How to Heal with
SINGING
BOWLS

TRADITIONAL TIBETAN HEALING METHODS

Third Edition

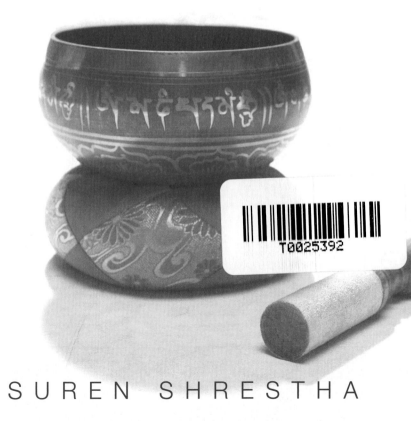

T0025392

SUREN SHRESTHA

To my father and mother, Surya Bahadur Shrestha and
Chhanda Shrestha, who gave me a positive outlook on life
and the inspiration to follow my dreams.

A paperback original

Cover design by Kim Johansen, *Black Dog Design*
Book design by Kim Johansen, *Black Dog Design*
Audio engineered by Daniel Mills, *Humble Sound Studios*

The information in this book is not intended as a protocol for the treatment of individual patients and is not a substitute for professional medical help.

Library of Congress Cataloging-in-Publication Data

Shrestha, Suren, 1966-
  How to heal with singing bowls : traditional Tibetan healing methods / Suren Shrestha.
— Third edition.
    pages cm
  ISBN 978-1-59181-287-6
  1. Singing bowl—Therapeutic use. 2. Healing—Himalaya Mountains Region. 3.
Traditional medicine—Himalaya Mountains Region. 4. Sound—Therapeutic use. 5.
Vibration—Therapeutic use. I. Title.
  RZ999.S542 2018
  615.8'5154—dc23
                        2018027780

Printed in the United States of America

10 9 8 7 6 5 4 3 2 1

Third Edition

SENTIENT PUBLICATIONS
A Limited Liability Company
PO Box 7204
Boulder, CO 80306
www.sentientpublications.com

Contents

Healing with More Than Two Bowls

Foreword

I RECENTLY had the very good fortune to attend a weekend course on the use of singing bowls given by Suren Shrestha, the author of this book. My partner, Aimee, had learned about the course from a mutual friend. I am a pediatric cardiologist, which means that I care for children with heart problems. Pediatric cardiology is a highly technical subspecialty. My training was based on Western scientific, linear, left brain experience and thought. Ten years ago, if anyone had told me that I would be open to using complementary medical practices, much less writing about them and promoting them, I would have told them they were crazy. But, here I am.

The shift began for me about ten years ago. After about eighteen years in practice, while experiencing the upside of Western medicine, I was becoming more and more aware of the downside. Patients undergoing surgery for congenital heart disease, with the accompanying stays in an intensive care unit, followed by protracted medical treatment and follow up, were developing other problems. These problems were resulting from their experiences with their disease and from the treatments for that disease. For example, babies who go through this process commonly develop gastroesophageal reflux. Oral defensiveness with incoordination of suck and swallow is also common. Older patients might have sleep disturbances, phobias, or difficulty maintaining focus in a classroom situation. Physical symptoms such as headaches, chest pain, palpitations and dizziness, in the absence of an actual cardiovascular cause, are common. Some develop anxiety or panic attacks with hyperventilation and its associated symptoms. More recently, some are being diagnosed with post traumatic stress disorder. These problems are often difficult to characterize accurately, and can be very difficult to treat.

A cardiologist faced with these issues will determine whether or not the symptoms have a true, organic cardiovascular cause. Very often, they do not. In that case, the patient is sent back to their primary care provider and from there perhaps to a gastroenterologist, pulmonologist, neurologist, or psychiatrist. Quite often, the patient never actually gets adequate treatment. The problems tend to persist, even if the patient develops improved coping mechanisms over time. Seeing more and more of this and not having anything terribly helpful to offer is very frustrating. I became more unhappy with these side effects as time went by.

I first became aware of CranioSacral Therapy a little over ten years ago. CranioSacral Therapy, or CST, is a gentle, noninvasive manipulative technique or modality. It uses very gentle maneuvers to basically remove obstacles that the normal, self corrective forces in the body have been unable to overcome. This practice incorporates mechanical, energetic, and intuitive means of diagnosis and treatment. It recognizes the whole individual, unavoidably leading to encounters with mind, body, and spirit as a continuum. CST can eliminate the problems I described above in most patients who have them. It does this gently and without negative side effects. It is economical, with no expensive equipment needed and no drugs to buy over periods of time.

Getting involved with CST opened a lot of doors for me. Not the least of these was openness to other complementary treatment modalities. Among these are sound and music therapy. The singing bowls might fall into this category. I am no expert on sound therapy, but I do have a feel for some of the theory behind the practice.

Everything is energy. How this energy behaves and what we call it depends on its rate of vibration and where we find it. This vibration is inherent in all things, and therefore, in all energy. The vibration may be at a very high frequency with relatively high energy, or it may be of a lower frequency with lower energy. This will be nothing new to most of you readers.

The term *entropy* refers to a degree of disorder. It is used to indicate disorganized energy. In a global sense, there is a tendency toward disorder, or we might say that the universe tends toward disorder or increasing entropy. However, locally, things tend toward energy equilibrium, or a higher degree of order. Using energy, we can locally decrease entropy, or increase the degree of order. A body tends toward order, not disorder. Trauma, or other pathology, might be looked at as a local area of increased entropy or disorder. It takes a certain amount of energy of a more harmonic nature, a higher degree of order, to decrease the entropy and to make things better. Reiki, CST, sound therapy, and other modalities might be seen as one person helping another to decrease the level of disorder in their body. Adding harmonic, organizing energy helps in this process. Sound is energy. Sound is vibration. Some of the most harmonic, beautiful, and effective sound that I know is produced by singing bowls.

During my weekend course with Suren, I was able to both treat and be treated with the singing bowls. Lying on a mat, surrounded by bowls of different pitches, I felt incredibly peaceful and relaxed, deeply meditative and content. The treatment always felt too short. With the bowls applied directly to the body, I could feel the sound go right through me. Tightness or resistance, along with any associated pain or discomfort, just melted away. We learned how to treat the whole patient in a number of ways, using different protocols. We also learned to use the bowls individually to focus on specific areas of the body. Suren Shrestha is a kind, intelligent, and spiritual man who has a talent for teaching.

There is a mounting body of experience, as well as research, that shows that meditation and sound therapies have a positive effect on actual measurable, identifiable anatomy and physiology. Sound can be a powerful aid in meditation itself. I am by no means the first or only Western style physician to open up to such ideas. An excellent case in point is Mitchell Gaynor, M.D. Dr. Gaynor is clinical professor of medicine at Weill-Cornell Medical College, and founder of Gaynor Integrative Oncology in New York City. He is also the author of *The Healing Power of Sound: Recovery from Life-Threatening Illness Using Sound, Voice, and Music* (Shambhala, 2002). Dr. Gaynor tells us that his success in treating patients with various forms of cancer has improved markedly since he began having his patients chant mantras while listening to the sound of singing bowls.

In my early work with CST, I first used it as an adjunct to my usual practice. As I gained experience and training, CST became more and more useful. Today, CST is my preferred approach to many problems seen in my patients. Of course, the patient always has a choice. When the choice is between a gentle, manual treatment that has no side effects, and a pill, they almost always choose CST. In these cases, CST is vastly more effective anyway.

I plan to use singing bowls in my practice, first as an adjunct to CST. However, I am sure that Suren and the bowls will show me more and more of what they can do, and that one day they will also assume a primary role in the treatment of many of my patients.

I am happy that Suren is sharing his knowledge with us in this book. As you read it, know that you are learning something of great importance and utility, and that you are learning it from a master.

—Andrew D. Fryer, M.D., F.A.A.P.

INTRODUCTION
What Is Sound and Vibration Healing?

EVERYONE has a vibration that is a signature of their health and wellbeing. You could think of it as a natural result of the processes that run our physical bodies as well as our mental, emotional, and subtle bodies. Similar to a musical instrument that can fall out of tune through use, our bodies can also fall out of vibrational harmony and potentially develop illness. Stress and negativity create blockages of a healthy flow of energy, showing up in the energy field around our body as lower energy disturbances at first, and later as illness in our physical body.

Sound and vibration can be used to re-tune us to health and one of the most powerful modalities for this is the use of Tibetan singing bowls. When there is a deep relaxation through soothing, resonant sound, the body is affected on a cellular level, opening up the flow of energy to move us back toward vibrational alignment with health. Sound can help us shift our energy frequency from lower to higher, removing the lower frequencies of emotions such as fear, anger, and resentment. In fact, whenever you are immersed in lower frequency emotions you can simply chant "Om" to elevate your energy.

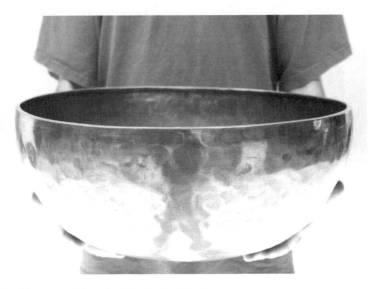

Hand-hammered twenty-inch singing bowl.

The sound of the bowls is calming, and they are frequently used as a meditation aid as the sound induces a sense of peacefulness.

Quantum physics has proven that everything has vibration, whether it's a table, a chair, a person, a planet, or a cosmos. And wherever there is a sound, there is a vibration. When we use sound coupled with intention, which is the most important aspect of healing, we can direct sound vibration to raise the body's vibrational frequency.

Negative energy can make us physically ill or mentally depressed. Each bowl emits a soothing vibration that radiates out negative energy, which restricts your ability to reach your full physical, spiritual, and mental health. Once your negative energy is radiated out through the vibration of the bowls, you're ready to allow yourself to live in healthy harmony with the immense energy of our seven creative planets.

Healing through sound and vibration has been known to reduce stress, improve concentration, reduce blood pressure, stimulate life force flow in the body, improve immunity, harmonize the chakras with the energy field, heighten intuition and perception, synchronize the brain hemispheres, remove mental and emotional negativity, and enhance creativity. Most importantly, stress is at the root of many of our twenty-first century diseases and it's through relaxation of the body that balance, health, and happiness can be restored. The salutary effect is produced by the unseen force of the vibrating bowls, combined with prayer. As much as 70 percent of the human body is made up of water, so when you strike a singing bowl next to your body, the vibration makes a mandala (a pattern) in your body, which is healing and relaxing.

How I Learned to Heal with Singing Bowls

Use of singing bowls for healing has been a dying art in Nepal. To my knowledge, only a handful of people in Katmandu and near the border of Tibet have been using them for healing. Chainpur and Bhojpour near my village of Khandbari, and the region near Katmandu, are the primary places where singing bowls and cooking utensils of metal alloy are made.

As far as my personal experience with the bowls, I grew up with metal alloy bowls used for eating or cooking. Though it was common to see bells of many sizes in the temples, even large hanging bells, it was not a common part of the Nepalese life to see singing bowls in the stupas, temples, and homes. Because my father came through a lineage of deep spiritual practitioners, I grew up with alternative healers such as shamans, monks, lamas, and bijuwas, and spiritual teachers such as pundits and gurus as a part of normal life.

Only in a handful of the healers' homes were singing bowls commonly found. The great teacher Master Dorje Tingo of Kimathanka is one of the healers I know who is actively using singing bowls for sound vibration healing in the traditional way. Another is Jejen Lama, who lives a two day walk from my village.

Just as with Thangka paintings, which are widely created by monks, lamas, Newar and Tamang clans, and many others, singing bowls are made by many people. However, there are few people making the singing bowls who practice the sacred chanting to infuse the bowls with healing intention.

Singing bowls are made in many countries. There are singing bowls from Japan known as rin gong, which are both machine made and handmade of metal alloy and are used mainly by Zen Buddhists for meditation. In Asia these bowls are often used for ritual purposes.

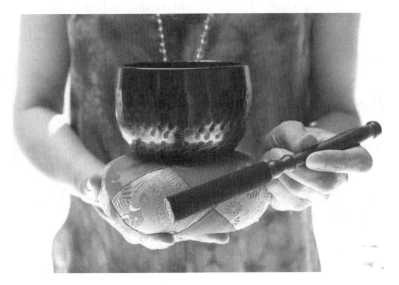

Japanese rin gong.

I want to clarify the name *Tibetan singing bowls*. The term is well known in western countries even though the bowls are native to the Himalayas, especially Nepal or India. In 1959, there was a large exodus of Tibetan monks to the west when the Dalai Lama left, and some brought their singing bowls with them, which they shared. I mention it here because it's widely understood that *Tibetan singing bowls* describes a type of hand hammered bowl from the Himalayas.

Since 1994, I have been actively studying traditional ways of healing with Tibetan singing bowls, traveling to Nepal sometimes twice a year to spend time with my teachers. The bowl layouts, mantras, importance of healing intention, and the therapies in my book represent what I have learned from my travels in Nepal. Some are from the Kimathanka region on the northern border next to Tibet. The knowledge of how to heal with Tibetan singing bowls is as old as the knowledge of how to make them. It has been handed down by the same verbal tradition and the same caste system that preserves the integrity of what is known through selection of one generational knowledge holder to the next, of which there may be many.

This body of knowledge is a gathering of practices from my many teachers, and according to all my teachers, you can integrate these methods into any therapeutic modality as long as the healing intention is present.

Why I Teach Healing with Singing Bowls

Growing up in Nepal, I learned about Ayurvedic healing because that was what was practiced there. We didn't have much Western medicine. I grew up in a culture where both Buddhist and Hindu practices were observed by most of the villagers, so it didn't matter which mantras, gods and goddesses, or religious holidays you observed. Prayer is an important part of using singing bowls for healing, but belief in a particular religion is not required. You can use your own faith, whatever it may be, to tap into the healing power of this art.

After I came to the United States as a young man, I realized that there was a lot of interest here in the ancient Eastern ways of healing. When I returned to Nepal, I started studying these techniques so I could teach them to people in the West. I have witnessed many people being helped through the use of singing bowls.

Because there is so much interest in these practices in the West, it is my hope that they will continue being used far into the future. It has became a fervent wish of mine to share my knowledge with people in these times when healing is so needed by everyone I meet.

Who This Book Is For

Whether you are a professional healer or you have never thought of yourself as someone with healing ability, you can use singing bowls to help yourself and others. In this book, I use the word *client* to describe the person who is receiving healing, but that doesn't mean you need to be a professional to use these techniques. Anyone with a clear intention and the willingness to learn how to use the bowls properly can create healing and relaxing effects in himself and others.

Using the Audio

You can download the audio file that accompanies this book at www.sentientpublications.com/singing-bowls-audio. It contains the following tracks:

1. Relaxation therapy
2. Chakra balancing therapy
3. Sound meditation

The first and second tracks are examples of two therapies described in this book. You can follow along with the audio, listening as I give the instructions before striking the bowls, and then strike your bowls at the same time as I do. Use the third track for meditation.

The History and Making
of Singing Bowls

THE MAKING of traditional singing bowls goes back some 2,400 years to the time of Buddha and has been handed down from generation to generation in India, Nepal, and Tibet through verbal teaching within a highly structured family clan or caste system. Today, craftsman in Nepal in the Kathmandu Valley work to revive the ancient techniques for making the bowls. The Shakyamuni clan today still makes healing bowls, chanting with mantras while they make the bowls. This is the same method that goes back to the time of Buddha.

The oral history tells us that the bowls came to Tibet from India at the same time that Buddhism was introduced to Tibet by the great Buddhist master Padmasambhava. Therefore, the history of Tibetan singing bowls goes back to the 8th century A.D.

These bowls are traditionally made of a special seven metal alloy of gold, silver, iron, mercury, tin, copper, and lead. Each of the sacred metals is aligned with the seven heavenly bodies in our solar system and the seven chakras of our body. Additionally, each bowl is fine tuned to the specific note that affects an individual chakra.

Each bowl begins as a molten mixture of the special seven sacred metals. It takes three to four people to hammer each bowl. One holds the hot metal with blacksmith tongs while two or three others alternate hammering and chanting, infusing the bowl with healing intentions even as it's being created. Bowls typically range in size from three inches to fourteen inches in diameter, but can also be larger or smaller.

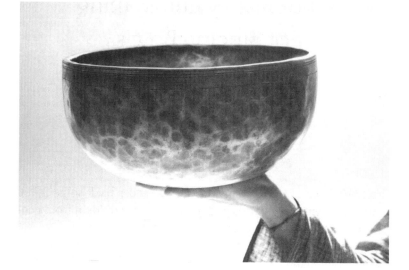

Antique hand-hammered bowl.

The Chakra Systems

SINGING bowls can open chakras, but this takes time. Chakras are energy centers in the body, corresponding to neural networks branching out from the spinal cord and glands in the endocrine system. When these centers are balanced, one's life becomes more balanced both physically, emotionally, and spiritually. Each chakra is associated with a note, color, seed mantra, body center, and various human qualities.

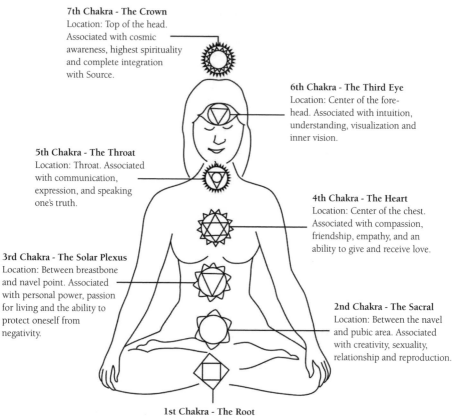

7th Chakra - The Crown
Location: Top of the head.
Associated with cosmic
awareness, highest spirituality
and complete integration
with Source.

6th Chakra - The Third Eye
Location: Center of the forehead. Associated with intuition,
understanding, visualization and
inner vision.

5th Chakra - The Throat
Location: Throat. Associated
with communication,
expression, and speaking
one's truth.

4th Chakra - The Heart
Location: Center of the chest.
Associated with compassion,
friendship, empathy, and an
ability to give and receive love.

3rd Chakra - The Solar Plexus
Location: Between breastbone
and navel point. Associated
with personal power, passion
for living and the ability to
protect oneself from
negativity.

2nd Chakra - The Sacral
Location: Between the navel
and pubic area. Associated
with creativity, sexuality,
relationship and reproduction.

1st Chakra - The Root
Location: Base of the spine.
Associated with issues of
survival, drive, ambition, and
grounding one's energy.

The seven chakras of the human body

The Vedic and Tibetan Chakra Systems

In the following charts, I give the Vedic and Tibetan systems for matching the chakras to notes, heavenly bodies, and metals. The two systems have evolved differently—you may choose which you prefer to use, or if you have a strong affinity to using a particular bowl for healing in a particular way, you can ignore both systems and use your intuition! If you feel, for instance, that the A bowl resonates with your heart, then perhaps you should use it for healing your heart. If you have only one bowl, you can certainly use it anywhere on the body. In this book, the therapies use the Tibetan system, because that's the way I learned.

Vedic System

Chakra	Vedic Note	Heavenly Body	Metal
7th - Crown	B	Jupiter	Tin
6th - Third Eye	A	Saturn	Lead
5th - Throat	G	Mercury	Mercury
4th - Heart	F	Sun	Gold
3rd - Solar Plexus	E	Mars	Iron
2nd - Sacral	D	Venus	Copper
1st - Root	C	Moon	Silver

Tibetan System

Chakra	Tibetan Note	Heavenly Body	Metal
7th - Crown	B	Moon	Silver
6th - Third Eye	E	Mercury	Mercury
5th - Throat	A	Venus	Copper
4th - Heart	D	Sun	Gold
3rd - Solar Plexus	G	Mars	Iron
2nd - Sacral	C	Jupiter	Tin
1st - Root	F	Saturn	Lead

The Tibetan order of planets corresponds to how fast they appear to move from the point of view of an observer on earth, with the moon as the fastest and Saturn the slowest, and the sun in the middle. This is an ancient system used by astrologers and alchemists, and of course, it doesn't include the planets that had not yet been discovered—Uranus, Neptune, and Pluto.

The System of Fifths

THE SOUND of the scale interval of a fifth is relaxing, soothing, and centering to listen to. Teachers of Tibetan singing bowl therapy from ancient times set up their singing bowls in a pattern where they strike the bowls in intervals of fifths because they feel this sound is beautiful to hear, and the vibrations of the fifth are especially good for balancing the heart chakra.

To arrange a set of singing bowls in fifths we simply set them up starting with F at the root chakra and go up five notes for each chakra.

Intervals	Bowl	Chakra
	F	Root
FGABC	C	Sacral
CDEFG	G	Solar plexus
GABCD	D	Heart
DEFGA	A	Throat
ABCDE	E	Third Eye
EFGAB	B	Crown

The old singing bowls from Tibet were made before modern tempered tuning entered into the stream of world music. The old bowls from Tibet often sound mysterious and multiphonic. Newer bowls made in Nepal in the last forty years are often more easily calibrated on an electronic tuner than the old bowls are.

Here is what a researcher in the field of harmonic vibrational theory—Dr. Harold Grandstaff Moses, director of the Institute of Harmonic Science in Phoenix, Arizona—has to say about the interval of a fifth:

> We have run numerous experiments with sound frequencies, harmonics, chord progressions, tempos, color, lighting and visual imaging in order to gain insight on ways to influence emotions and feelings, while facilitating healing, reducing stress and generating a heightened state of spiritual awareness. Our research indicates that the musical interval of the perfect fifth (a mathematical relationship of 3:2) and the resulting harmonic overtones have the ability to favorably influence the parasympathetic nervous system while modifying the listener's state of consciousness.
>
> I am fascinated by the approach to the chakra system through a map based on perfect fifths. I encourage any soundworker to experiment with this tuning system. Certainly there is room for a re-evaluation of existing theories in light of the new discoveries which are being made regarding the uses of harmony for healing.

How to Buy a Singing Bowl

DIFFERENT bowls correspond to different chakras, and produce different notes on the musical scale. You can choose a bowl that is appropriate for the particular kind of healing you want to do. For example, you may want to become more compassionate, so you could use the F bowl in meditation to open your heart chakra. For healing, you would use the D bowl to affect your heart chakra.

The best way to choose a bowl is to play different bowls until one of them feels right to you. The bowl will speak to you and you will know that is the one you need. The sound will be soothing and relaxing to you. Don't choose a bowl by the way it looks but by the effect the sound has on you. Rubbing and striking give you different tones—try both. You really should hear the bowl before you buy it.

Crystal singing bowls are also available, but these are not the traditional singing bowls discussed in this book.

There are bowls that are made of three, four, five, seven, and even nine metals. Most machine-made singing bowls are less than seven metals, and are mainly used for meditation. When selecting bowls for healing purposes, seven-metal bowls are preferred.

Bowl Size

Large bowls have stronger, deeper vibrations. Small bowls have higher, more intense vibrations. The human body responds differently to sounds in the higher or lower octaves of sound. Some people find that they prefer the sound of the bigger bowls with their lower pitch and deep low vibrations.

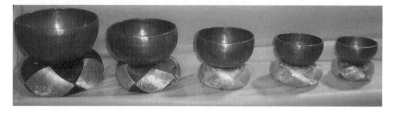

Four-inch to ten-inch bowls.

Starting Out

You may want to buy your first bowl for personal healing. If you purchase one large bowl (around 8-14") you will be able to use it for all the personal healing therapies. You may also want to buy a smaller singing bowl (3-7") for use in meditation. For those who are prepared to jump in a little faster, consider getting up to four bowls at first. A healing bowl costs at least two or three hundred dollars and can be as much as two thousand dollars for the antique ones. You could start by buying a smaller, inexpensive meditation bowl, which you should be able to get for about twenty-five dollars, and then work your way up.

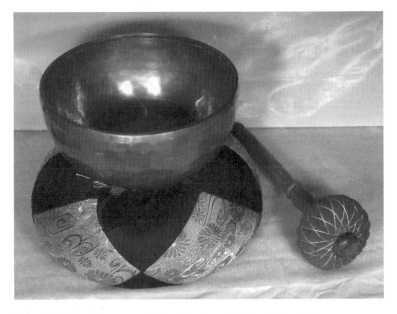

Seven-inch hand-hammered Nepalese bowl with velvet mallet.

Choosing a Bowl Based on Sound

When choosing a single singing bowl, first play it with a felt or leather mallet and listen to the quality of the resonance and of the tone of the bowl. Strike the bowl again, and now hold the top lip of the bowl 2-3" away from your mouth while opening and closing your mouth. This should easily produce a "wah-wah" sound effect, which is a desirable technique. When I am trying out a bowl I play it with a leather or wooden mallet to hear if the song around the side of the bowl is smooth and steady. If it's a big bowl I try it on my head and play it to see the quality of the sound.

Make sure one note predominates. In the event that the bowl is multiphonic, with more than one note, then choose the longest note to define your bowl. You may find it useful to use a note finder (an electronic tuner) to accurately identify the note of the bowl.

If the bowl has a crack in it, it can be very hard to see, but you can tell by listening to the sound whether it has been damaged.

Sometimes a cracked bowl no longer resonates when struck, giving instead a dull metallic clunk sound. Or, if it's a hairline fracture that's difficult to see, you may hear an annoying rattle or buzzing sound. Sometimes, in spite of the crack or even a hole in the bowl, the bowl still resonates. Regardless, a damaged singing bowl should not be used for healing or even for meditation. Instead, return the bowl to the dealer or store so they can send it to their manufacturer for recycling.

Buying a Set of Singing Bowls

If you're thinking of buying a set of bowls matched to the seven chakras, buy them all together if you can, as you will want to hear them as a set. If you're ordering them wholesale ask the seller to make a set for you. Be sure you know whether you are buying a bowl that is handmade or machine made.

It's best to sit down with many bowls and put your set together at a location where you can listen to a variety of bowls. Often a shop will let you return a bowl that is too large or too small or that has a tone you no longer enjoy, if you have a relationship with that shop. Your assessment of a bowl may change after you start working with it. Your apprehension of pitch will tend to become very discerning once you are absorbing the sound of your set of bowls every day. People often want to trade bowls for reasons of pitch or bowl size or the configuration of the different size bowls within the set.

If you're buying a set of bowls and you start with a bowl that has a sharp tone, you may want the F, G, A, C, D to all be sharps. If you start with naturals you may want all the notes to be natural. This isn't a rule, but it does help consider the harmonic relationship.

Some people say that for concerts the bowls should be very harmonically pleasing to listen to. For a healing set this isn't so important. When putting together a set of bowls for healing it helps if you lie down with the bowls around you and listen to them and feel their vibrations.

Some say that you shouldn't break up a set once you have put it together and are satisfied with it. The bowls will sing together when the energy is good.

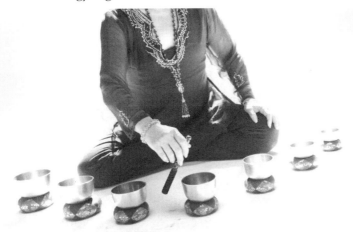

Set of seven smaller bowls.

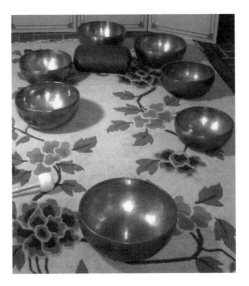

Set of seven larger bowls.

Caring for Your Bowls

USE HALF a lemon and warm water to wash the bowl—never use brass polish. Play the bowl each day to honor your relationship with it. If you are going to put the bowl on the body you should put warm water in it to balance the elements (earth, air, fire, water, metal).

When you travel with singing bowls, wrap them in newspaper, cloth, or bubble wrap so that they don't rattle and bang into each other. You can nest the smaller bowls in the bigger ones as long as you protect them from each other by wrapping. You can carry them in a suitcase or heavy canvas bag.

Playing the Bowls

YOU CAN play a singing bowl by rubbing or striking it. Striking gives you a clearer tone and rubbing gives a stronger vibration. Sit in a relaxed position with your back straight, on a chair or cushion on the floor. Your eyes should be relaxed and slightly closed. If you are right-handed, hold the bowl on the palm of the left hand (vice versa if you are left-handed) at the level of your heart. Keep the hand that is holding the bowl flat—don't curl your fingers around the bowl or they will impede the sound. Take a deep breath and think only of your breathing as you begin to play. Strike the bowl with an upward stroke, except when the bowl is upside down, in which case you use a downward striking motion (for example, when the bowl is placed on the head).

Rubbing the Bowl

Use either a wooden or a leather covered mallet. With leather you get a softer tone, while wood gives you a higher pitched sound. Using a wooden mallet is a good way to learn, because it's easier to

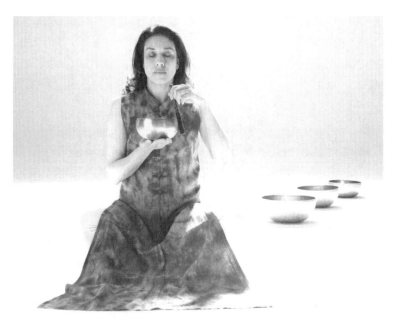

Seated posture for playing a singing bowl.

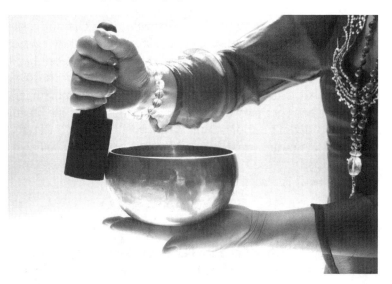

Rubbing the bowl for meditation.

get a sound. With a leather mallet, you have to press a little harder, but there's no rattling sound.

For Meditation

Place the bowl on your flat palm and move the mallet slowly in a clockwise direction. If the bowl is too large or heavy to fit on the palm of your hand, you can place it on a table or cushion. Traditionally, you do not combine hitting the bowl with rubbing for meditation purposes. Do not use the wrist, but instead use the movement of the elbow and shoulder to move the mallet around the outside mouth of the bowl, keeping the whole mallet in constant contact with the bowl. If you begin to create a rattling sound, this is not desirable—slow down.

For Healing

You can place the bowl directly on the body if it's three to fourteen inches in diameter. The bowl can also be placed on a table or the floor. Use three fingers (ring, middle, and index) on the inside center of the bowl to stabilize it as you rub the bowl with the mallet.

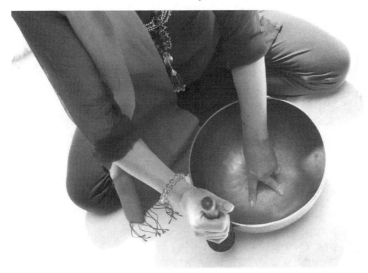

Rubbing the bowl for healing therapies.

To initiate the vibration, you can strike the bowl gently and then rub the mallet back and forth from right to left to bring out the bowl's healing vibrations.

Striking the Bowl

Make sure you strike the bowl with an upward motion of the striker (except when otherwise noted). A common mistake people make when first learning to play a singing bowl is to tap it rather than using a fluid upward stroke.

For Meditation

Use either a leather, brocade, or felt covered mallet. Place the bowl in the palm of your hand, or on a cushion, the floor, or an altar table. Strike the bowl

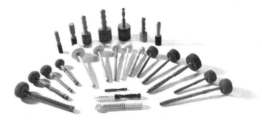

Rubbing and striking mallets.

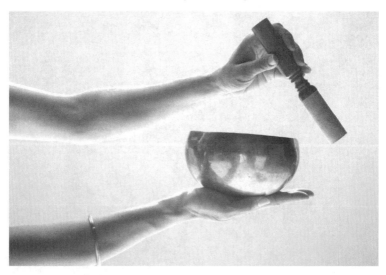

Striking the bowl for meditation.

and move the mallet upwards at the end of the stroke's path. This creates a golden, resonant, vibrating tone.

Listen to the subtle, soothing sound vibration of a single strike as you inhale, following the sound of your breath as the sound dissipates to silence. You may also strike three times as you begin your meditation. Continue your meditation into the silence. End your meditation with a single strike.

For Healing

Use either a brocade-covered or felt-covered mallet. You can place the bowl directly on the body, on the floor, or on a healing table.

On the body, use three fingers (ring, middle, and index) on the inside center of the bowl to stabilize it if the bowl is small.

On the floor or on a table, place the bowl on a non-slip pad to prevent the bowl from shifting. You can make your own pads from soft, non-adhesive material made for lining kitchen drawers and shelves.

Begin the strike from three feet out and make contact one inch below the rim of the bowl. At the end of the stroke's path, move the mallet upward to create a full and resonant tone. You may hit the inside upper rim of the bowl, still making an upward sweep at the end of the stroke's path. To initiate the vibration, you can strike

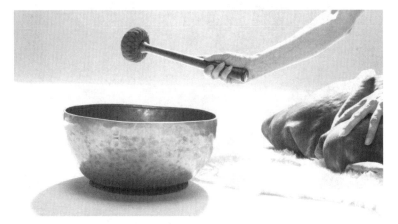

Swinging the mallet for healing therapies.

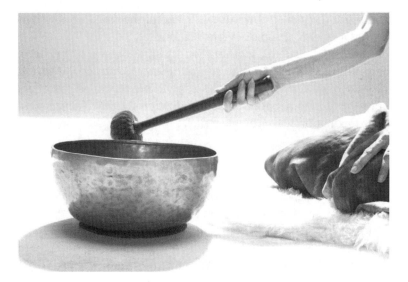

Striking the bowl for healing therapies.

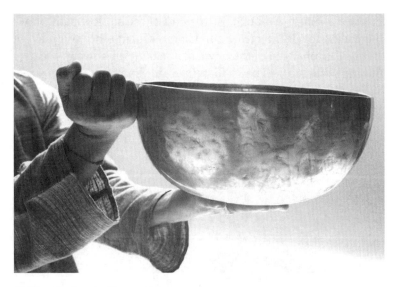

Striking the bowl with your fist.

the bowl gently and then rub the mallet back and forth from right to left to bring out the bowl's healing vibrations.

Striking the Bowl with Your Fist

Hold a large bowl in your non-dominant hand. Make a fist with your other hand and strike the bowl near the rim with the little finger side of your fist to make a gentle and soothing sound. This is used most often in the healing therapies where a softer vibration is desired.

Playing the Tingsha

The tingsha is made up of two small metal gongs connected with a leather strap. The best way to play the tingsha is to hold the strap close to the metal, holding one side of the tingsha in each hand. Turn one gong so the striking edge runs vertically, turn the other so the striking edge runs horizontally, and bring them together to make the sound.

Traditionally, the tingsha has been used to make music, to clear negative energy from a space, and to bring the mind into the present moment. It has also been used to heal tinnitus. Spiritually, the tingsha has been used to open up the inner vision of the third eye. It's also used to create a healing connection to share the positive energy between the healer and the client. And, finally, the tingsha is used to balance the chakras.

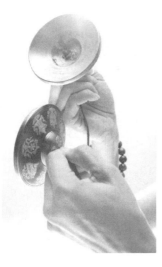

Playing the tingsha.

Bell and Dorje

The bell is the only instrument I have seen played in temples during services. The purpose of the bell is to awaken you to the present moment. I use it in pujas (prayer services) and meditation, but not in healing therapies. You can hit the bell with a wooden mallet, or you can simply ring it.

The dorje is made out of metal or crystal and is in the shape of two ovals joined by a smaller ball, with a shaft running through them. Dorje means thunderbolt in Tibetan. It's also sometimes described as a diamond scepter and is a sacred symbol of wisdom. People use it in meditation, holding it in one hand in a mudra position. The bell is held in the left hand and the dorje in the right—together they represent feminine (bell) and masculine (dorje).

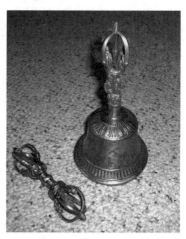

Bell and dorje.

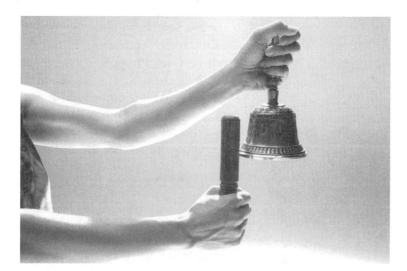

Ringing the bell.

Setting up the Environment

THE ENVIRONMENT in which you provide healing and meditation for yourself or others should be a quiet, clean, orderly, uncluttered, and pleasing space. All the information in this section applies whether you are giving yourself or someone else a treatment. A carpeted floor may be comfortable for lying on, but the bowls will resonate better on a hard surface, so you can make the client (or yourself) comfortable on a mat if you are using a room with a wooden or tile floor. Wood is an especially good surface for transmitting the vibrations.

You will need a small pillow for the client's head, and many clients like small pillows under their knees when they are on their backs. Your client will be more relaxed if you cover her eyes with an eye pillow or a dry wash cloth. If you use an eye pillow, cover the eyes with a clean tissue before applying the pillow, for sanitary reasons. Similarly, use paper towels over the pillows for the head and knees, so that each client gets a clean surface. The pillows should be made of natural materials.

The best lighting is dim, and if you can use candles to light the space it creates a pleasing effect.

Make sure that the room is warm enough for the client, who will be lying motionless for quite a while and can easily become cold. You can place a light blanket over the client if necessary.

The room should smell nice, or at least not have an unpleasant odor! You can burn incense or a scented candle prior to the healing session, but be aware that some people are very sensitive to any kind of smoke or scent, so always ask before you prepare the room.

If you use water in the bowls it should be very warm, not scalding hot. *Do not pour hot water into a bowl while it's on the client's body.* Before placing the bowl on the client, test the temperature by placing it on your own skin. If it's too hot, add some cool water. Be especially careful when placing a warm bowl on the third eye chakra, the palms, or naked feet. It's best to use an electric kettle to keep the water warm and keep cool water nearby in case you need it.

The client should wear loose fitting, natural fiber (cotton is best) pants and a shirt. If you have an altar table, a statue of a god or goddess, or a picture of a revered being in the treatment room, then the client's head should point toward it.

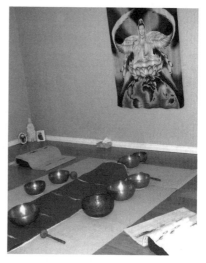

A healing environment.

Group Meditation

Sometimes I join with other singing bowl practitioners to create a group meditation, where the meditators lie on the floor with a blanket and pillow, sit in chairs, or sit on cushions while the meditation leaders play the bowls, bells, gongs, and tingsha. This provides a wonderful relaxing environment for people to use whatever meditation practice they prefer. The following photograph shows how bowls can be set up for such a group meditation.

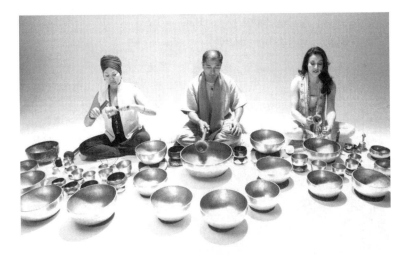

Leading a group meditation.

If meditators lie on the floor, their heads should be oriented toward the bowls.

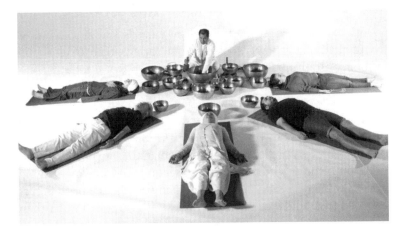

Positioning of meditators.

Using a Singing Bowl Sound and Vibration Healing Table

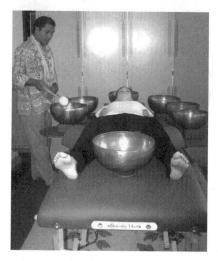

For westerners it's sometimes difficult to perform singing bowl therapies on a client lying on the floor. It can be hard on the knees and back of the healer. A good alternative is to use a healing table, such as the one that I've designed, shown in the following photograph. You could also use a massage table and place the bowls on stools or standing TV trays. You may need a cushion under the bowls to raise them to a height level with the table.

Singing bowl sound and vibration healing table.

Safe Practices When Using Singing Bowls

Although food is served from metal utensils and in some cases from actual singing bowls in Nepal, it isn't appropriate to serve food in them or to drink from them in the western world today.

ADD and ADHD as well as other conditions where a person may feel excitable or hypersensitive are best worked with by playing the singing bowls quietly and slowly, and by placing them farther away from the person's body.

It is inappropriate for a pregnant woman to be exposed to loud noise on or near her belly. I do not recommend playing singing bowls on the belly of a pregnant woman because the baby is surrounded by a fluid world. Sound travels faster through water than through air so the effect would be to speed up the vibrations. So, if you want to give a singing bowl treatment to a pregnant woman, place the bowls a few feet from the body and play gently.

Using Your Intuition

THIS IS A how-to book, so I give instructions here for the way I generally practice these healing therapies. However, I rarely do exactly the same thing more than once. I vary the treatment depending on the client's particular needs, and my intuition about what will work best. So, I encourage you to do the same!

I learned many different techniques from a variety of teachers and I choose from these therapies what I feel is appropriate in a particular circumstance. Please feel free to modify anything you learn here to suit your own needs or your client's.

If you trust your intuition, you will allow the unseen healing force that is all around you to be expressed naturally. This is where the true healing comes from—you can't *really* do it "by the book"!

Personal Healing Therapy

THE FOLLOWING therapies can be done on yourself or on others. Any time a bowl is placed on the body it can be done with or without warm water in the bowl.

NOTE: I use the words *she* and *he* to describe clients simply to avoid more awkward wording, however all the therapies are appropriate for both male and female clients.

Healing with One Bowl

First and foremost, you choose a chakra bowl based upon what feels soothing to you, what resonates with you. Use this bowl for healing any part of your body. Remember that your intention is an integral part of this modality. You are capable of healing yourself, so open your intuition as to where you should place the bowl. You can use this one bowl on the heart, tummy, solar plexus, thigh, knee, or calf. If you are a healer working with just one bowl, you can also use the bowl on the client's back, shoulders, legs, and feet.

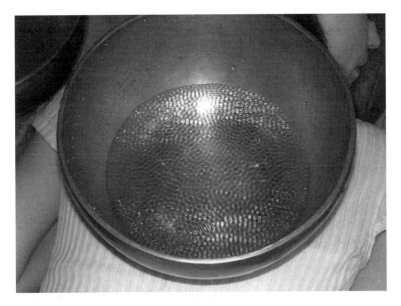

Using water in the bowl.

You can enhance this technique by filling the bowl one quarter full with warm water, which will cause the healing vibrations to penetrate more deeply into the body.

Clearing the Chakras with Seed Mantras

Use this personal healing method to remove negativity and blockages of specific chakras. In order to heal chakra imbalances, you need to be in a quiet, private space where you will not be disturbed for the length of the treatment. If you have only one bowl, use that bowl to clear your chakras. If you have a set of chakra bowls, then use the bowl that corresponds with the chakra you wish to clear.

Sit in a comfortable position, either on a chair with both feet on the floor or on a cushion with your legs crossed, or sitting on your heels. Sit with back erect, chest out and up, shoulders relaxed and parallel to the ground, chin pulled back one inch. You can either close your eyes, rolling them in and up to the third eye, or you can

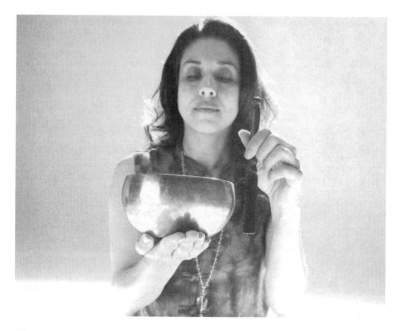

Clearing the chakras with seed mantras.

leave the eyes nine-tenths open, gazing at the tip of the nose. Both eye positions stimulate the intuition of your third eye.

Center yourself and follow the breath. On the inhale, bring your attention to the issue or specific chakra with the intention to clear negativity and to heal. On the exhale, release all that does not serve your highest needs, sending the negativity down your legs, out the soles of your feet, and to the core of the earth, where it will be broken down into elements to be reincorporated into new life.

If you're sitting in a chair you can either hold the singing bowl in front of your heart or you can place it on a table in front of you. If you're sitting cross legged on the floor, hold the bowl on your open palm at your heart. Now either strike or rub the bowl.

Concentrate on your breath and connect with your emotion. Gradually draw your attention to your chakra point(s) and chant the seed mantra for that particular chakra. You can do this for as long as you desire or until you feel the release of the negativity. Feel the emotion without judgment and dwell in the present moment.

Chakra	Vedic Note	Vedic Mantra	Tibetan Note	Tibetan Mantra
7th Crown	B	Silent	B	Silent
6th Third Eye	A	Om	E	Aa
5th Throat	G	Ham	A	Om
4th Heart	F	Yam	D	Hung
3rd Solar Plexus	E	Ram	G	Ram
2nd Sacral	D	Vam	C	Dza
1st Root	C	Lam	F	Silent

Healing the Head

Approximately 7 minutes

This is an effective treatment to release stress after a day of hard work at the office or after any activity that causes tension to build up. One of my teachers, Dorje Thingo, showed me this alternative method of healing to cure insomnia, migraine headaches, and muscle tension.

This personal healing therapy can be done while sitting on a cushion or on a chair. First, place either a towel or a piece of non-slip cushion liner on your head to stabilize the bowl. Then invert a large bowl and place it on the top of your head. Be sure it's balanced and comfortable! Then gently hit the bowl with a downward striking motion. Wait twenty seconds and repeat, gently. Be sure to practice quite a bit with the bowl on your head, making sure you can balance it. If the bowl were to fall, it could hurt you or hurt your bowl, so take precautions.

You can create a deeper relaxation and healing effect by making a vibration sound chamber that brings two bowls into a reciprocal sound relationship. To do this, the first bowl is placed on your head as above, and the second is held in your non-dominant hand. Hold the second bowl in the palm of your hand between your heart and solar plexus. The size of your second bowl will determine how high you will raise it after striking. If the bowl is similar in size to the one on your head, then raise it up to your throat chakra after striking. If the bowl is between 4 and 8" in diameter, raise it up to your third eye chakra after striking. Regardless, hold the bowl at the ending place for a few moments and repeat as desired.

If a healer is assisting you, have him hold the second bowl 2-4" away from your throat chakra and gently hit the bowl with two upward striking motions. As the bowl he's holding vibrates, he should move it slowly downward in a Z motion from the throat to the sacral chakra, and then from the sacral chakra, he should raise the bowl straight even more slowly up to the crown chakra. You may repeat this as many times as you like.

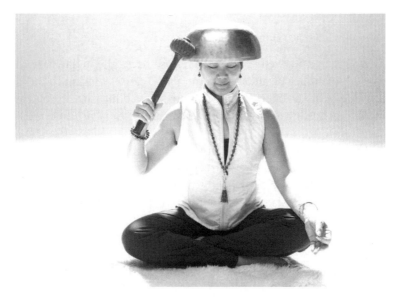

Healing the head using one bowl.

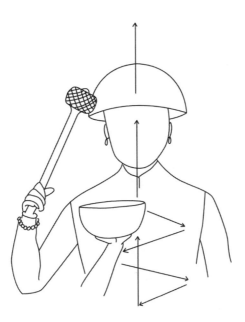

How the healer moves the second bowl

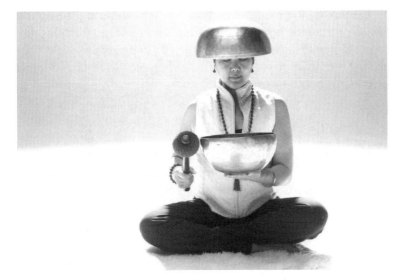

Healing the head using two bowls.

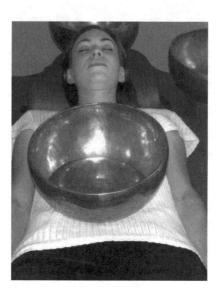

Healing the front of the body.

Healing the Front of the Body

Lie down on a mat or a bed and lay a bowl on the area to be healed. Strike the bowl gently upwards and let the vibrations dissipate for ten to fifteen seconds. As the vibrations play, inhale deeply, feeling the vibrations in your body, and on the exhale clear out any pain. Repeat as long as needed.

Healing the Feet

Sit in a chair or stand and place your bare feet in the middle of a large bowl. If the bowl isn't large enough to fit both feet in it, you can tip your feet so either the top or the back of your feet are in contact with the bowl. Strike the bowl gently upwards and let the vibration dissipate for ten to fifteen seconds. As the vibration plays, breathe in deeply, feeling the soothing sensations, connecting through the reflexology points to all the parts of your body. Repeat as long as needed.

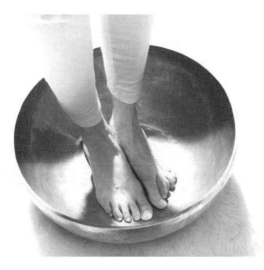

Healing the feet on your own.

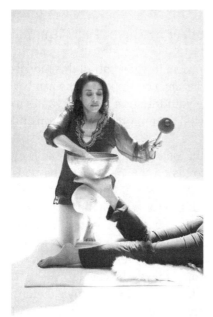

Purchasing a bowl large enough to fit both feet into (around 18") is rather expensive as the bowls are very large and heavy. To get around the price issue, you can have a healer assist you with an 8-14" bowl placed on the sole of your foot. Rest your foot on the healer's knee and have her strike the bowl as described above.

A healer works with the feet.

Healing Therapies for Clients

THE FOLLOWING therapies are done by a healer for a client. You cannot do these on yourself.

Remember that your intention is an integral part of this modality. The intention, thought, and belief are most important. Remember, too, that you are capable of using your intuition to guide you as to where you should place the bowl(s) to support the relaxation and healing of your client.

Each time you place a bowl on the client's body, precede it by placing your hand for a few seconds on the area where the bowl will rest, avoiding, of course, any sensitive areas. For example, the heart and root chakras are close to private areas of the body, so be aware of where you place your hand. Focus your healing intentions through the touch of your hand. There is a brief transfer of healing touch as your hand is quickly but gently replaced by the bowl, so that the change is almost unnoticeable to the client.

In the role of healer, you may decide to employ a single therapy for a sixty minute session. However, you also have the option of customizing a sequence of therapies from the following list to meet

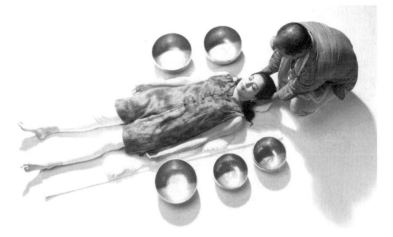

Cradling the client's head.

the unique needs of your client:

- Healing with one and two bowls
- Relaxation therapy
- Chakra balancing
- Warm water therapy on the front of the body
- Healing prayer
- Warm water therapy on the back

Opening and Closing a Healing Session

The setting of healing intentions is begun by the healer at the opening of the session. You may use any words or prayers that come from your background of healing. It is important that your earnest energy is focused for the highest good of all. This is done in two steps. First, focus on the breath to come into a deep state of emptiness (shunyata). Then, when the mind is cleared, focus your highest intention (sankalpa or will) on the client's healing. This helps the healing energy penetrate to the client. Having a clear mind attunes and harmonizes the mind and body.

Getting to shunyata, you may experience many thoughts flowing into your mind, but do not be concerned. Regard these thoughts with no more concern than if they were bubbles popping out and clearing, bringing you closer to the state of pure emptiness. It can take time, but be patient and you will be rewarded. Once you experience shunyata, you can more easily flow your intentions to the area where the client needs healing because you have cleared your mind of outside concerns.

You may ask the client to express her healing goals as well, either silently or out loud. If she mentions that a particular part of her body or an emotional issue needs healing, then concentrate your energy on that throughout the session. At the start, tell the client what to expect and how to make the transition at the close of the session. For example, you may tell her that at the end you'll quietly leave the room and then she can take her time, or you could give her some time limit for resting before she arises.

To begin the therapy itself, cradle the client's head gently with healing intention, breathing deeply while giving energy through your touch. (If you are trained in cranial-sacral massage, use your technique at this point.) After holding the client's head for a minute or two, turn your palms downward and slowly sweep your hands to the sides of the client's head, releasing the client's negative energy.

Next go to the client's feet and cross your hands so your right hand is lightly touching their left foot, and vice versa with your left hand. You may massage the feet while sending energy. After holding the client's feet for a minute or two, turn your palms downward and slowly sweep your hands to the sides of the client's feet to ground the client's energy.

At the closing of the session, provide the client with a glass of water and remind her to drink plenty of fluids throughout the day.

Healing with One or Two Bowls

One or two bowls can be used for healing any part of your client's body. Choose a bowl or bowls based upon what feels soothing to you and resonates with you.

If you are working with just one bowl, you can use it on the client's back, shoulders, legs, feet, or wherever your intuition leads you. If you're using two, you can place one each on any pair of these areas: the heart, solar plexus, thigh, knee or calf.

Some Techniques for Using One or Two Bowls

- Hold one offering-style bowl (about 6 inches in diameter) flat on your palm or perched on your fingertips, and play the bowl by rubbing or striking.
- Focus on the area you want to heal: physical, emotional, mental or spiritual.
- Smaller bowls are especially useful for working with the mind. The mind controls the body and the healing vibrations cascade into the body through the mind's avenues. Larger bowls are required to physically penetrate deep into the body with the vibrations.
- You can use one large bowl for all chakras; you can work on the entire body using just one or two bowls.
- When the client is lying on their stomach, a good technique is to place one bowl (especially a smaller one) above the head and one on the back.
- The longer you wait between striking the bowls, the more grounding it is.
- Augment the healing treatment by filling a bowl to be placed on the client's body with warm water. This will cause the healing vibrations to penetrate more deeply into the body. The bowl should be filled to less than one quarter of its volume. After pouring the warm water into the bowl, hold the bowl in both hands and bless the water. This is very important because it helps to set the intention for the healing.
- Using mantras in combination with singing bowl vibrations increases positive healing energy.

Healing with One Bowl

In these first two techniques you will be working directly with the aura, or energy body. Etheric energy is a type of fine matter that surrounds us and permeates all that is physical. Some refer to it as chi, universal life force energy, or prana. In physics, it's described as a wave-and-particle type of energy, and it affects everything in our physical and emotional universe.

Clearing the Aura, or Energy Body

Approximately 3-5 minutes

The client can be in a variety of positions, such as standing, sitting or lying down.

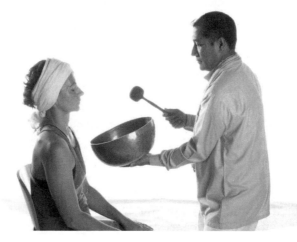

Clearing the aura.

Small Bowl – 4-8" Diameter

1. Hold the bowl in one hand and start by striking or rubbing the bowl softly with a leather-covered striker, which will give a soft vibration. Strike the bowl away from the client, then bringing it to about 5-6" from their hairline to avoid creating disturbance.

2. Pause the bowl and then slowly move it in a clockwise direction around the client's head.
3. Completing a circle, pause again at the hairline and then move the bowl straight up to about 1 foot above the head and pause there until the vibration dissipates.
4. Repeat steps 1-3 twice, for a total of 3 times.

Larger Bowl – 9-14" Diameter

Clearing the aura can be done with the smaller bowl, as described above, however, it is more effective to use a larger bowl because of its deep resonance. The heavier weight will require that you use more strength to hold it, so take that into account. With larger bowls, use a fist strike or mallet strike, since rubbing is difficult.

Clearing the Chakras

Approximately 3-5 minutes

The client can be in a variety of positions, such as standing, sitting or lying down.

Allow your intuition to direct you in moving the bowl from front to back, side to side, or around the body.

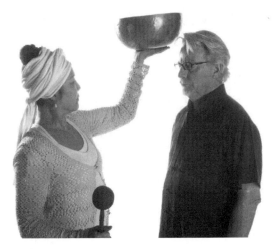

Clearing the chakras.

Small Bowl – 4-8" Diameter

1. Hold the bowl in one hand and start by striking or rubbing it softly with a leather-covered striker, which will give a soft vibration.
2. Strike the bowl away from the client, bringing it in toward their body to avoid creating disturbance. Bring the bowl up to the hairline and pause.
3. Then slowly move down through the third eye, throat, heart, solar plexus, sacral, and root chakras.
4. The sound will be dissipating by the time you reach the root chakra, so strike it again at this point and then move up slowly through the chakras and back to the hairline, then pause again.
5. Finally, move the bowl straight up to about 1 foot above the head and pause there until the vibration dissipates.

One Larger Bowl – 9-14" Diameter

Clearing the chakras can be done with the smaller bowl, as described above, however, it is more effective to use a larger bowl because of its deep resonance. The heavier weight will require that you use more strength to hold it, so take that into account too. With larger bowls, use a fist strike or mallet strike, since rubbing is difficult.

Treatment for Insomnia

Approximately 10 minutes

The client may be in a sleeping position for this treatment, lying on their side with a bolster between their legs, or perhaps lying on their back with a bolster under their knees, whatever is most comfortable for the client. It's very effective to use a larger bowl, such as one 10" or more in diameter, however, a smaller, 4-6" bowl can be used as well. The larger the bowl, the deeper the vibration, and thus, the deeper the relaxation. Chanting Om in unison with the bowl's note is very effective as well.

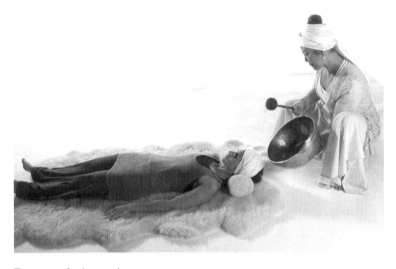

Treatment for insomnia.

1. Hold the bowl in one hand a couple of feet away from the client and start by striking it with the side of your fist or the mallet to produce a deep vibration. If the bowl is too heavy to hold for the whole treatment, you can make an adaption to the healing setup. If you're treating a family member, they can scoot down in the bed so the bowl can be placed on the bed above the head, on a singing bowl cushion. This is a specially constructed cushion for the bowl, which prevents dampening of the bowl's healing vibrations. If the client is on a massage table, ask them to place their head below the face cradle. Then the bowl can be played on the singing bowl cushion on top of the face cradle. If you're using a small bowl, you can hold it on the palm of your hand or perched on the fingertips and strike it softly with the mallet.
2. Then bring the bowl to a position 3-4" above the client's crown chakra and hold it there until the vibration completely dissipates.

3. Wait another 30 seconds in the silence to promote Theta brain waves, which accompany a deeply meditative state. This period of complete silence is important to the effectiveness of the treatment.

4. Before striking the bowl for the next repetition, move it 2 feet away from the client's head once more, strike, and then move the bowl back into position 3-4" above the crown chakra and hold it there until the vibration dissipates.

5. Repeat steps 1-4 at least 5 times.

Treatment for Shoulder, Neck and Upper Back Tension
Approximately 7-10 minutes

For this treatment, the client can be sitting on a chair or comfortably seated on a cushion on the floor. However, the most effective setup is to cradle the client's face in the face cushion of a traditional massage chair because the angles of the shoulders, neck and cranial areas will be optimal. Rest the bowl on the cranial-sacral area, where the neck and the skull come together.

To maximize the healing effects, it's best to pair a 10-12" diameter bowl with a 2-3" diameter leather rubbing mallet. This produces a deeper healing vibration from the bowl, penetrating the body at the cellular level.

Place the bowl on the client's shoulder, holding it in place with the fingertips of one hand inside, pressing the bottom of the bowl in such a way that the bowl can be rotated to deeply massage and penetrate the tissues of the body as it is vibrating.

Continue rubbing the bowl as you move it across the client's neck, upper back, and other shoulder.

Healing with Two Bowls

Note that the two bowls you use can be of any notes as long as they are different.

General Relaxation and Healing Therapy
Approximately 25-30 minutes

Recommended sizes for the two bowls in this therapy are 4-8" for the smaller one and 9-12" for the larger one. The smaller bowl will be played with a .75 to 1.5" diameter leather-covered mallet and the larger bowl with either a 1.5 to 3" leather-covered rubbing mallet or a fabric-covered striking mallet. Deeper healing vibrations result when rubbing the bowl, however striking with the mallet is still good.

For the first part of this therapy, the client lies on his back, either on the floor or a massage table, with his arms resting at his sides and his legs together.

As you grow in your skill you can advance to using warm water inside the larger bowl in this technique. However it's best to keep the water level less than one quarter of the bowl's volume to prevent it from splashing out onto the client.

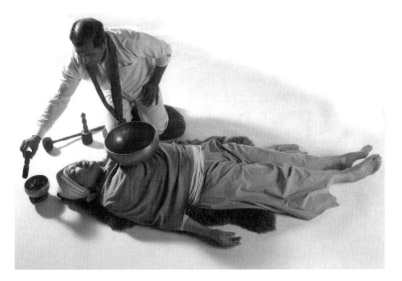

General relaxation and healing therapy: striking the smaller bowl when treating the front of the body.

Treating the Front of the Body

1. Place the larger bowl 3 to 4" from the crown of the head.
2. Strike the bowl 3 times softly at intervals of 5 seconds. After the third strike, wait for 20 seconds or until the sound almost completely dissipates. It's important to strike the bowl as softly as possible to avoid jarring the client's healing state.
3. Place your hand on the client's forehead (third eye) and then slowly remove it while replacing it with the smaller bowl. **Gently** strike it 3 times at 5 second intervals and then wait 20 seconds or until the sound almost dissipates.
4. When there is a deep state of emptiness or shunyata in the silence, strike the larger bowl 3 times as described in step 2 above.
5. To treat the throat chakra, place the smaller bowl high on the chest, making sure the edge of the bowl doesn't touch the chin. Or, you may place the bowl directly on the client's chin. Gently strike it 3 times at 5 second intervals and then wait 20 seconds or until the sound almost dissipates. Repeat this sequence 2 times. In the silence of shunyata, strike the larger bowl 3 times as described in step 2 above.
6. When the vibrations of the larger bowl dissipate, replace it with the smaller bowl, so the smaller bowl now sits 3-4" above the crown of the head. Put the larger bowl on the side for the moment.
7. Strike the smaller bowl 3 times softly at intervals of 5 seconds. As the vibrations from the final strike dissipate, place the larger bowl on the heart chakra.
8. Strike the larger bowl 3 times softly at intervals of 5 seconds. If you are an advanced practitioner you can follow this by rubbing the larger bowl with the leather-covered mallet for 1 to 2 minutes to apply deeper healing vibrations. You can do this for each step below in which you strike the larger bowl on various parts of the body. If you

are not using the rubbing technique, after the third strike, wait for 20 seconds or until the sound almost completely dissipates.

9. Repeat step 7 above, but this time move the larger bowl to the solar plexus chakra as the vibrations from the final strike dissipate.

10. Strike the larger bowl 3 times softly at intervals of 5 seconds. If you follow this with the rubbing technique, keep in mind that the softness of the abdomen may make it harder to achieve an effective healing vibration. Sometimes you can fix this by rubbing at a slightly faster speed. If you are not using the rubbing technique, after the third strike, wait for 20 seconds or until the sound almost completely dissipates.

11. Repeat step 7 but this time move the larger bowl to the sacral chakra.

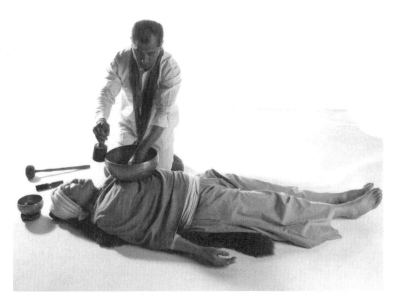

General relaxation and healing therapy: rubbing the larger bowl when treating the front of the body (advanced).

12. Strike the larger bowl 3 times softly at intervals of 5 seconds. After the third strike, wait for 20 seconds or until the sound almost completely dissipates.
13. Repeat step 7 but this time move the larger bowl to the upper root chakra. The proper placement of the larger bowl will be just at the top of the pubic bone area.
14. Repeat step 7 to complete this part of the treatment.

Treating the Thighs and the Calf of the Lower Leg

1. When working on the legs you may find it easier not to alternate between the smaller and larger bowls, because the greater distance between the legs and the crown makes it difficult. Or, if you have another person working with you, they can continue the alternate striking of the smaller bowl at the crown described in step 7 of the section above.
2. Place your hand on one of the client's thighs and slowly remove it while replacing it with the larger bowl. Rub for a minute, or strike 3 times, waiting 5 seconds between strikes, and then wait 20 seconds, until the sound almost dissipates. Repeat with the other thigh.
3. Place the larger bowl on the calf of one leg to the side of the shin bone and rub or strike 3 times, waiting 5 seconds between strikes, and then wait 20 seconds, until the sound almost dissipates. Repeat with the calf of the other leg. (With a larger client it may be easier to change the sequence and complete the thigh and calf on one leg and then move to the other.)
4. As an advanced technique you can complete this section by striking or rubbing the larger bowl as it is simultaneously rotated and moved through the chakras on the front of the body, down to the thighs and lower leg. Start from the heart chakra, strike and wait 5 seconds as you rotate and slide the larger bowl to the next chakra, etc.

Treating the Back of the Body

1. Gently ask the client to turn over on their tummy.
2. Place the smaller bowl on the floor or table 3-4" above the crown chakra. Strike it 3 times, pausing 5 seconds between the first two strikes. After the third strike, wait for 20 seconds or until the sound almost completely dissipates. Strike the bowl as softly as possible to avoid jarring the client's healing state.
3. This step works with the larger bowl to heal the third eye from the back of the head. Hold the larger bowl in one hand and strike it with the small finger side of the fist of your other hand, or with a felt covered mallet. Move the vibrating bowl from the left side of the head to the right side, 3-4" from the body, in an arc shape that traces along the Occipital Ridge (the region at the back of the head where the base of the skull meets the spine). Repeat this 3 times. Each time, strike the larger bowl at 20 second intervals, or until the sound almost dissipates.
4. When there is a deep state of emptiness or shunyata in the silence, repeat step 2 above.
5. Place the larger bowl behind the throat chakra, at the neck and upper shoulder part of the back. Strike the bowl 3 times, waiting 5 seconds between strikes, and then wait 20 seconds, until the sound almost dissipates. Repeat step 2 above.
6. Place the larger bowl on the heart chakra and strike 3 times, waiting 5 seconds between strikes, and then wait 20 seconds, until the sound almost dissipates. Repeat step 2 above.
7. Repeat the individual instruction for the large bowl followed by step 2 as you move down the remaining chakras until you reach the root chakra. You'll move through solar plexus, sacral and root chakras. When working on the lower body you may find it easier not to alternate between the smaller and larger bowls, because the greater distance

between the legs and the crown makes it difficult. Or, if you have another person working with you, they can continue the alternate striking of the smaller bowl at the crown described in step 2.

8. Place the larger bowl on the buttock and strike 3 times, waiting 5 seconds between strikes, and then wait 20 seconds, until the sound almost dissipates. Repeat step 2 above. Repeat with the other buttock.

9. Place the larger bowl at the back of the thigh and strike 3 times, waiting 5 seconds between strikes, and then wait 20 seconds, until the sound almost dissipates. Repeat step 2 above. Repeat with the other thigh.

10. Place the larger bowl at the back of the knee and strike it 3 times, waiting 5 seconds between strikes, and then wait 20 seconds, until the sound almost dissipates. Repeat step 2 above. Repeat with the other knee.

11. Place the larger bowl on the calf and strike it 3 times, waiting 5 seconds between strikes, and then wait 20 seconds, until the sound almost dissipates. Repeat step 2 above. Repeat with the other calf. (With a larger client it may be easier to change the sequence and complete the buttock, thigh, knee, and calf on one side and then move to the other.)

12. Advanced practitioners may rub the larger bowl for about one minute after striking in each chakra position while moving through the steps of this therapy. The vibration from rubbing the bowl is very effective.

Treating the Soles of the Feet and Palms of the Hands

1. Bend the client's leg and place their foot on your thigh or on a bolster. Then place the larger bowl on the sole of the foot and strike 3 times, waiting 5 seconds between strikes, and then wait 20 seconds, until the sound almost dissipates. In this step the healing energy moves up the client's leg. Repeat with the sole of the other foot. (Advanced

practitioners may choose to rub the bowl for 30 seconds to 1 minute after striking, waiting about 20 seconds for the vibrations to dissipate before moving on in both this step and step 2.)

2. Place the larger bowl on the palm of the client's hand and strike 3 times, waiting 5 seconds between strikes, and then wait 20 seconds, until the sound almost dissipates. To balance the bowl on the palm, it may help to place a folded washcloth under the client's hand. In this step the healing energy moves up the client's arm. Repeat with the palm of the other hand, and when the vibration completely dissipates, wait another minute or two at the conclusion of this treatment.

Deep Double Rub - Advanced Therapy
Approximately 15-20 minutes

This is a very advanced method and you should be well along in your practice before undertaking this with your clients. It involves rubbing two bowls simultaneously, which requires good coordination. Usually people find it easiest to rub both bowls in the same direction—either clockwise or counterclockwise. This therapy uses heated herbal pads placed directly on the body, so you must take care that they are not so hot that they will burn your client. The bowls are then placed on top of the pads so the vibrations are combined with the heat to deeply penetrate into the body.

This treatment is easy to do on a massage table, but it can also be done on the floor. It is given either on the front or the back of the body (or both), and regardless of which side of the body you choose to work on, the instructions below are the same.

You will need:
- Two 9-12" diameter bowls of any two different notes. Each bowl must have a non-slip pad underneath to keep it from sliding off the heated herbal pads.
- Two 1.5-2" diameter leather-covered rubbing mallets. Each is

10-11" in total length with the leather coming 5-6" up the length of the mallet.
- Two 4-7" diameter heated herbal pads of ¼" thickness. These will be placed directly on the body underneath the bowls. Lavender or any herbal combination for relaxation is recommended.

1. Heat the two herbal pads in the microwave to the desired temperature, making sure that it is comfortable on your own skin.
2. Place one of the bowls on its non-slip pad 3-4" above the crown of the client's head. If you are using a massage table, place the bowl on the face cradle on top of a singing bowl cushion that will prevent the bowl vibrations from being dampened by the face cradle's cushioning.
3. Place the other bowl and one of the herbal therapy pads on the client's heart chakra. Note, the placement will consist of several layers of material in the following order, starting closest to the body:
   - Heated herbal therapy pad
   - Non-slip pad (same diameter as the singing bowl)
   - 9-12" diameter singing bowl
4. With one leather-covered mallet in each hand, begin by rubbing the crown bowl for 1-2 minutes.
5. Continue rubbing the crown chakra bowl as you begin rubbing the heart chakra bowl simultaneously for 1-2 minutes. This will result in the crown chakra receiving 2-4 minutes of vibration while the heart chakra receives 1-2 minutes. Allow the vibrations to dissipate.
6. Move the crown bowl and its non-slip pad from its original position. Place it onto the client's body at the sacral chakra (lower abdomen). Use the same placement order of materials as noted in step 3 above. However, the softer abdominal tissue can make it difficult to vibrate the bowl. In that case, try placing the bowl on top of the pubic bone, which can make it easier to vibrate the bowl.
7. Rub the heart chakra bowl for 1-2 minutes. Continue

rubbing it as you also begin rubbing the sacral chakra bowl simultaneously for another 1-2 minutes. This will result in the heart chakra receiving 2-4 minutes of vibration while the sacral chakra receives 1-2 minutes. Allow the vibrations to dissipate.

8. Finally, move the heart chakra bowl and its non-slip pad and herbal therapy pad to the spot in between the legs just above the knees, if the client is on his back. If the client is on his stomach, the bowl setup will be on the back of the knees.

9. Rub the sacral bowl for 1-2 minutes. Continue rubbing the sacral bowl as you begin to simultaneously rub the bowl on the knee/thigh for another 1-2 minutes. This will result in the sacral chakra receiving 2-4 minutes of vibration while the thighs/knees receive 1-2 minutes. Allow the vibrations to dissipate and gently remove the bowls from the client.

Modified Baby Posture

Approximately 10-15 minutes

This therapy stimulates the aura, or energy body. The client's head, chest, abdomen and hips rest lengthwise on two bolsters stacked on top of each other. Her head is turned so her cheek rests comfortably, her elbows rest on the floor, and her hands loosely hug the front of the bolsters. Eyes are closed. This posture makes her back fairly level, so that you can place the bowl on it. This therapy can be done with one or two bowls. Stand or kneel to either side of the client.

You will need:

- Two bolsters, 31" long x 14" wide x 9" high
- Optional massage table
- One or two 8-12" diameter bowls of any note
- One large fabric-covered striking mallet
- One 1.5-3" diameter leather-covered rubbing mallet

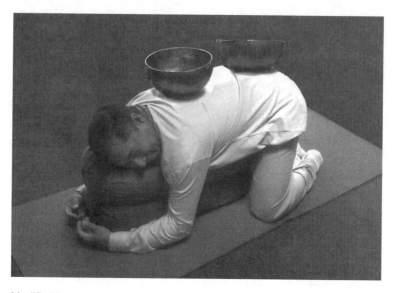

Modified baby posture.

1. Gently place one hand at the small of the back.
2. Stand or kneel in a grounded position and feel your weight resting equally throughout your body. Relax your jaw, face, and shoulders. Take 3 long breaths to center yourself, and bring your awareness to your contact with the client. Establish a rapport with the client's internal bodily rhythm. This step may take 2-3 minutes.
3. Place a bowl where your hand was and strike it 3 times in rapid succession. Wait until the vibrations almost dissipate, then rub the bowl for about a minute. Allow the vibration and sound to dissipate.
4. If you're using one bowl, slowly remove the bowl and bring it to the shoulder region. Gently place a hand in between the shoulders and then replace the hand with the bowl. Strike it 3 times in rapid succession. Wait until the vibrations almost dissipate, then rub the bowl for about a minute. Allow the vibration and sound to dissipate.

5. If you're using two bowls, you will leave the first one on the small of the back and place the second between the shoulders using the healing touch before placing the second bowl. Strike the second bowl on the shoulders 3 times in rapid succession. Then wait until the vibrations almost dissipate and rub the bowl for about a minute. Allow the vibration and sound to dissipate. Note: You won't be using the bowl at the small of the back.

6. If you're using one bowl, repeat steps 1, 3 and 4 for a total of 3 repetitions.

7. If you're using two bowls, repeat steps 3 and 5 for a total of 3 repetitions. Note: After the first repetition, the bowls will be in place at the small of the back and at the shoulder region so you will just be striking and then rubbing the bowls as specified in steps 3 and 5.

8. Remove the bowl(s) and have the client lie on her back in the yoga dead pose for 2 minutes or more, so that the body can integrate the sound vibrations it has received. While the client is lying down, place your hands on either side of her head, with fingers flanking the ears. Center yourself by breathing deeply. Take 3 long breaths in and out, and bring your awareness to where your hands are touching her head. Relax your jaw, face, and shoulders. If you're standing, align your body in a grounded position with both feet solidly on the floor. If you're sitting, feel your weight resting equally on your sit bones. Note any changes in what you feel as you touch the client. You are looking for changes in the quality of the tissue, to see if it has softened and become more resilient. The client's breathing should also have slowed down and deepened. These are indications that the body is responding to the power of the sound vibration.

Healing with More Than Two Bowls

Relaxation Therapy

Approximately 15 minutes

Relaxation therapy balances blood circulation, producing a relaxation response.

Positioning the Client and Placing the Bowls

Ask the client to lie on his back on the floor with legs apart. His arms and hands can be by his sides or on his tummy. For the client's comfort, have pillows nearby to place under his knees. You can sit by the client's hip on either the right or left side. Place the bowls

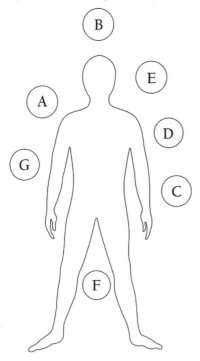

as indicated in the following drawing and photograph.

In this therapy, the bowls do not touch the body, so before beginning, check the positioning of the singing bowls to verify they are within two to four inches of the body, but not touching the client's body or other materials that would dampen the bowl vibrations. Each bowl position should be level with the corresponding chakra location. The bowl you place by the third eye chakra should be more than six inches from the client's head.

**Bowl placement for
relaxation therapy**

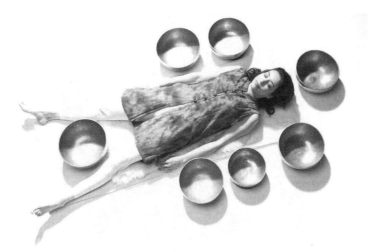

Positioning the client for relaxation therapy.

Striking the Bowls

When striking a multi-note bowl sequence, pause five seconds between each of the bowls in the sequence. Though pause times can be shortened to meet a time schedule, keep in mind that the duration of the bowl vibrations greatly enhances the healing effects of this therapy. After the final bowl in a sequence is played, pause twenty seconds before beginning the next sequence.

Part 1: Relaxing

# of Bowls	Tibetan Notes	Repetitions	Sequence Pause Time
4	BFDG	3	20 seconds
5	BFDGC	1	20 seconds
4	BFDG	3	20 seconds
6	BFDGCA	1	20 seconds
4	BFDG	3	20 seconds
3	CAE	1	20+ seconds until no sound

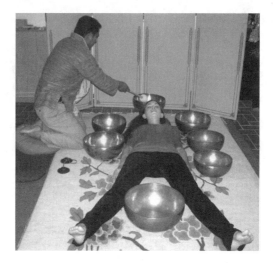

Striking the B bowl.

Part 2: One-by-One

# of Bowls	Tibetan Notes	Repetitions	Sequence Pause Time
7	BEADGCF	1	20+ seconds until no sound

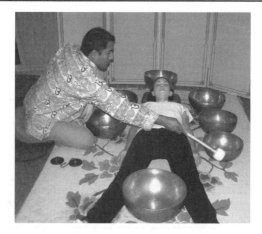

Striking the C bowl.

Part 3: Reverse

# of Bowls	Tibetan Notes	Repetitions	Sequence Pause Time
7	FCGDAEB	1	20 seconds
2	FB	1	20 seconds
2	DG	1	20 seconds
3	CAE	1	20+ seconds until no sound

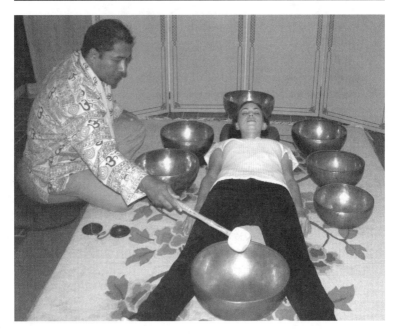

Striking the F bowl.

Additional Technique for Inducing Tranquility in the Mind

When you set up the bowls for the relaxation therapy, you may include a set of seven smaller meditation bowls placed around the client's head, as in the following photograph. These can be used during the therapy to create a more tranquil mind.

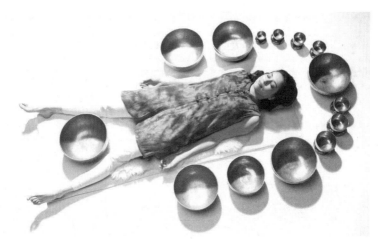

Bowl placement for inducing tranquility in the mind.

After you complete part 2 of the relaxation therapy, softly strike the third smallest bowl, the second smallest, and then the smallest bowl in rapid succession. If you strike the bowls too hard, you will induce something other than tranquility! Wait until the sound is nearly dissipated before softly striking the second largest, third largest, and fourth largest bowls without pausing in between. When the sound dissipates, strike the largest bowl, the second smallest, and the fourth largest bowl, waiting 5 seconds between bowls. Then continue with part 3 of the relaxation therapy, and repeat this sequence with the small bowls at the end.

Healing Prayer

Approximately 7 minutes

In this therapy you will chant and use the bowls to direct energy to whatever the client is experiencing as a problem area in their body/mind. This therapy provides removal of blockages to activate healing.

Positioning the Client and Placing the Bowls

Ask the client to lie on her back on the floor with legs apart. Her arms and hands can be by her sides. For the client's comfort, have pillows nearby to place under her knees. You can sit by the client's hip on either the right or left side. Place the bowls as indicated in the following photograph.

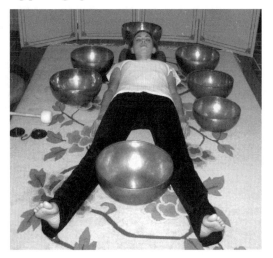

Placement of bowls for healing prayer therapy.

Part 1: Preparing for Healing

Place the **C** bowl on the **sacral chakra** and proceed to play the bowls. (Placing the C bowl on the sacral chakra is an optional step—use your intuition as to whether this is appropriate for your client or not. If you decide against it, just leave the bowl in its usual position.) Pause five seconds between each bowl in each of the two multi-note bowl sequences.

# of Bowls	Tibetan Notes	Repetitions	Sequence Pause Time
7	BFDGCAE	1	20 seconds
7	FBDGCAE	1	20+ seconds until no sound

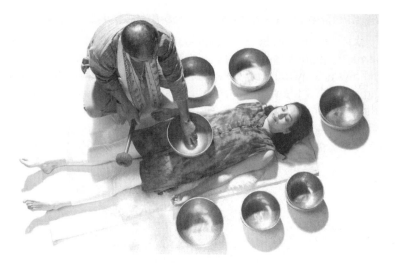

Playing the C bowl on the sacral chakra.

Part 2: Healing Prayer

# of Bowls	Tibetan Notes	Repetitions	Sequence Pause Time
7	FCGDAEB	1	Immediately play the small bowl

Immediately play a 4-6" bowl 2-3" above the **third eye** by striking the bowl with a felt or leather covered mallet or by rubbing the bowl with a wooden or leather covered mallet. Slowly move the bowl in a clockwise upward direction while chanting a healing mantra from your heart. Choose a mantra that is appropriate for your client's condition. A prayer from your own faith may also be used. If you'd like to use the Vedic mantras as part of this Tibetan therapy, it's fine to mix the two cultures!

These are the Vedic mantas:

- The seed mantra for the root chakra is Lam (rhymes with *mom*)
- The seed mantra for the sacral chakra is Vam (rhymes with *mom*)

- The seed mantra for the solar plexus chakra is Ram (rhymes with *mom*)
- The seed mantra for the heart chakra is Yam (rhymes with *mom*)
- The seed mantra for the throat chakra is Ham (rhymes with *mom*)
- The seed mantra for the third eye chakra is Ohm (rhymes with *home*)
- The seed mantra for the crown chakra is silence

This is where unseen force comes up for the healer. You may feel sensations or movement coming through your body. This is the time to ask your teachers, guides, ancestors, god, to assist in directing the healing energy to come in through your crown chakra and move it out through your third eye chakra to heal the client. Focus all your energy into the movement of this unseen force to the client for healing in the physical, emotional, or spiritual realms of their life.

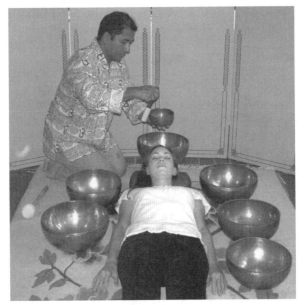

Striking the bowl above the third eye.

Mantras for Healing the Chakras

When chanting a mantra to heal a chakra, vibrate the mantra in the head and chest to penetrate deeply.

Muladahara

- 1st chakra: the root chakra
- Issues: material world, safety, finances, home life, groundedness
- Physiology: low back, legs, lower sexual organs, adrenals
- When out of balance, anger is felt.
- The seed mantra LAM balances this chakra through vibration.

Svadisthana

- 2nd chakra: the sacral chakra
- Issues: feelings, emotions, sexual energy, creativity
- Physiology: uterus, ovaries, large and small intestines, spleen
- When out of balance, addictive behavior, depression, anxiety, or detachment from feelings is common.
- The seed mantra VAM balances this chakra through vibration.

Manipura

- 3rd chakra: the solar plexus chakra
- Issues: will, need to control, self esteem, self worth
- Physiology: stomach, pancreas, liver, gall bladder, spleen, kidneys
- When out of balance, control issues, low self esteem and criticism of others can occur.
- The seed mantra RAM balances this chakra through vibration.

Anahata

- 4th chakra: the heart chakra
- Issues: expression of virtues such as love, compassion, kindness, forgiveness
- Physiology: heart, lungs, thymus

- When out of balance, energy will be directed toward lower chakras. In order to conduct the higher energy of the higher chakras opening the heart center is imperative. The heart is the center of communication with divinity.
- The seed mantra YAM balances this chakra through vibration.

Vishudda

- 5th chakra: the throat chakra
- Issues: expression of energy through speech, ability to connect with others through verbal expression and with divinity through prayer
- Physiology: throat, thyroid, parathyroid, ears, sinus
- When out of balance, the other chakras have no means of releasing energy.
- The seed mantra HAM balances this chakra through vibration.

Ajna

- 6th chakra: the brow chakra, or the third eye
- Issues: clairvoyance, spiritual center, images in the mind, psychic awareness, meditation
- Physiology: pituitary, eyes, autonomic nervous system
- When out of balance, energy will be directed toward the self rather than to service to humanity or earth healing.
- The seed mantra Om harmonizes with divine energy through vibration.

Sahaspara

- 7th chakra: the crown chakra
- Issues: oneness with all, harmonious, peaceful, loving, non reactive, non-attached
- Physiology: top of head, pineal gland
- When out of balance, guidance will not be received from divine energy through this chakra and energy will not descend to the lower chakras.
- The seed mantra is silence, no sound.

Balancing the Chakras

Approximately 10-12 minutes

This therapy opens the third eye chakra energy, promoting understanding of inner vision. Once the third eye is open, negative energy gradually dissipates, grounding you from negative influences both internally and externally. Therefore, the chakras are equalized and balanced. This therapy has been found to help with high blood pressure, depression, stress, and insomnia.

Positioning the Client and Placing the Bowls

Ask the client to lie on her back on the floor with legs apart. Her arms and hands can be by her sides or on her tummy. For the client's comfort, have pillows nearby to place under her knees. You can sit by the client's hip on either the right or left side.

In this therapy the bowls again do not touch the body. Remove the **C**, **E**, and **A** bowls and place them off to the side. You may reverse the positions of the **B** and **F** bowls and repeat parts 1-3 for another ten minutes to accommodate your client's need for more extensive chakra healing work. Place the bowls as indicated in the following photograph.

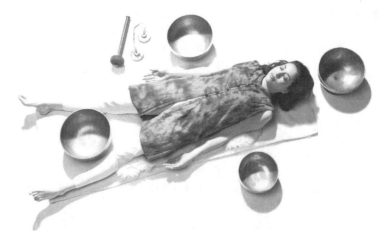

Bowl placement for chakra balancing therapy.

Part 1: Share Heart to Heart Healing Energy

The purpose of part 1 is to create a healing energy creation between the client and the healer.

# of Bowls	Tibetan Notes	Repetitions	Sequence Pause Time
2	BF or FB	1	5 seconds
2	DG	3 times quickly	1-2 seconds

During the vibrations of the bowl sequence, play the tingsha as follows. Place the tingsha about a foot away from your heart chakra and play it. Then as it is ringing, turn the concave side of the tingsha toward your heart and move it in to a position about 4 inches from your heart. Then, as it rings, move it in to about 2-4" from the client's **heart**. Then move the tingsha as follows:

- to the client's **throat chakra**
- to the client's **third eye chakra**
- to the client's **sacral chakra**
- retrace back to the client's **throat chakra**
- to the client's **third eye chakra**
- and finally, to your **heart chakra**

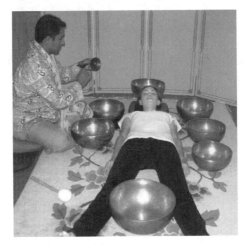

Moving the tingsha from the healer's heart to the client's heart.

Part 2: Opening the Third Eye Chakra

The purpose of part 2 is to awaken your intuition.

# of Bowls	Tibetan Notes	Repetitions	Sequence Pause Time
2	BF or FB	1	10 seconds
2	DG	3 times quickly	1-2 seconds

During the vibrations of the bowl sequence, play the tingsha. Start one and a half feet above the client's **third eye**, then move quickly to one inch over the **third eye**. Move the tingsha while the bowls are playing to the **throat chakra** and then to the **sacral chakra**. Retrace back to the **throat chakra** and then to the **third eye chakra**. Slowly raise the tingsha up to one and a half feet from the **third eye** until the sound of the tingsha dissipates.

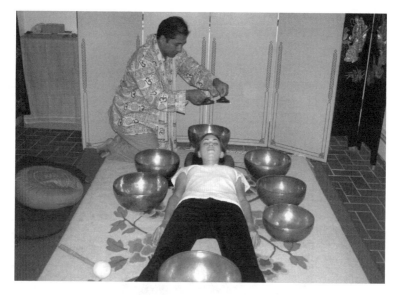

Playing the tingsha over the third eye.

Part 3: Balancing the Chakras

The purpose of part 3 is to create balance and harmony between the chakra centers.

# of Bowls	Tibetan Notes	Repetitions	Sequence Pause Time
2	BF or FB	1	10 seconds
2	DG	3 times quickly	1-2 seconds

During the vibrations of the bowl sequence, play the tingsha. Start one and a half feet above the client's **sacral chakra**, move quickly to one inch over the **sacral chakra**. Move the tingsha while the bowls are playing to the **throat chakra** and then to the **third eye chakra**. Retrace back to the **throat chakra** and then to the **sacral chakra**. Slowly raise the tingsha up to one and a half feet.

Warm Water Therapy

Approximately 15 minutes

When you use warm water in the bowls, the water helps to transmit the positive energy of the vibrations of the bowls to the client. Don't forget that the water should be very warm, not too hot. Before placing the bowl on the client, you should test it on yourself. If necessary, you can add some cool water. Take extra care when placing a water-filled bowl on the third eye, the palms, or naked feet. You can use an electric kettle to warm the water and keep some cool water nearby.

Positioning the Client and Placing the Bowls

Ask the client to lie on his back on the floor with legs apart. His arms and hands can be by his sides. For the client's comfort, have pillows nearby to place under his knees. You can sit by the client's hip on either the right or left side. Place the bowls as indicated in the following photograph.

Check the positioning of the singing bowls to verify they are within two to four inches of the body, but not touching the client's

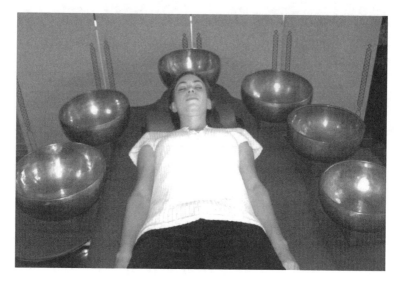

Bowl positioning for warm water therapy.

body or other materials that would dampen the bowl vibrations. Each bowl position should be level with the corresponding chakra location. The bowl you place by the third eye chakra should be more than six inches from the client's head.

Fill an 8–10" bowl one-quarter full with warm water. Choose a bowl according to the note that is appropriate for your client. This bowl will be placed onto the body during the following multi-note bowl sequences. To hold the water-filled bowl on the body, rest your fingertips inside the bowl, spread out on the bottom. You may have to tilt the bowl slightly to balance it.

Part 1: Warm Water Therapy on the Front

THERAPY FOR THE FIRST LEG

# of Bowls	Tibetan Notes	Repetitions	Sequence Pause Time
7	BEADGC	3 times softly	20+ seconds

After striking the sequence above, place the warm water bowl on the client's lower shin (either left or right) and strike the bowl three times quickly. Let the vibration dissipate 10-20 seconds. Then move the bowl up the leg to the shin, avoiding the bone, and strike. Next, place and strike above the knee. And finally, place and strike on the upper thigh.

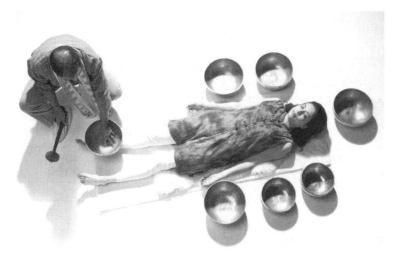

Placing the water-filled bowl on the client's leg.

THERAPY FOR THE SECOND LEG

# of Bowls	Tibetan Notes	Repetitions	Sequence Pause Time
7	BEADGC	3 times softly	20+ seconds

Repeat the sequence above and then place the warm water bowl on the other shin and continue up that leg as described above. You may make additional placements as you move up the leg if desired. As an alternative to striking the bowl, you may use a rubbing technique, which brings the healing deeper.

THERAPY FOR THE FIVE CHAKRAS

# of Bowls	Tibetan Notes	Repetitions	Sequence Pause Time
7	BEADGC	3 times softly	20+ seconds

Place the water-filled bowl on the following 5 chakras—sacral, solar plexus, heart, lower throat, and third eye. Strike the bowl softly 3 times, letting the sound dissipate.

Part 2: Warm Water Therapy on the Back

Before beginning, remove the **F** bowl and ask client to turn over onto her stomach. She may need to remove the pillow.

THERAPY FOR THE FIRST LEG

# of Bowls	Tibetan Notes	Repetitions	Sequence Pause Time
6	BEADGC	1 time softly	20+ seconds

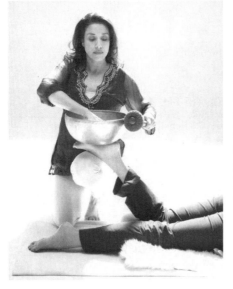

After striking the multi-note bowl sequence above, place another water-filled bowl on the foot of the first leg (see the following photograph for placement) and strike 3 times quickly, letting the vibrations slowly die down (10-20 seconds). Then move the bowl up the leg striking 3 times in each position.

Bowl placement on the foot for warm water therapy.

THERAPY FOR THE SECOND LEG

# of Bowls	Tibetan Notes	Repetitions	Sequence Pause Time
6	BEADGC	1 time softly	20+ seconds

Repeat the sequence above and then place the water-filled bowl on the remaining foot and continue up that leg as described above. You may make additional placements as you move up the leg if desired. As an alternative to striking the bowl, you may use a rubbing technique, which brings the healing deeper.

THERAPY FOR THE SPINE AND SHOULDERS

# of Bowls	Tibetan Notes	Repetitions	Sequence Pause Time
6	BEADGC	1 time softly	20+ seconds

Strike the multi-note bowl sequence above, placing the water-filled bowl on the tail bone as you strike the first note (B) of the sequence. This makes a gentle transition for the client.

Then strike the water-filled bowl three times quickly and let the vibration dissipate 10-20 seconds. You'll move the bowl a few inches up along the spine each time and in each new position you'll strike the bowl three times quickly and then let the vibrations dissipate for 10-20 seconds. As an alternative to striking the bowl, you may use a rubbing technique which brings the healing deeper.

Once you've reached the top of the spine, you can massage the entire back by first hitting the bowl, then rotating it back and forth approximately 90 degrees while moving it across the shoulders and down to the lower back. This sends the vibrations deep into the muscles where they can penetrate and relax tension. You can massage all over the back as needed with this technique. Then bring the water-filled bowl back to the tail bone where it will rest for the remainder of this therapy and play it regularly whenever the sound dissipates.

Repeat the multi-note bowl sequence **BEADGC** above, periodically in this section of the healing therapy if you like.

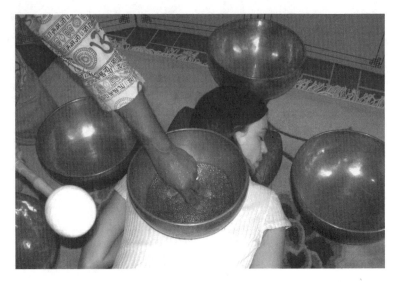

Placing the water-filled bowl on the back.

CLOSING THE SESSION

# of Bowls	Tibetan Notes	Repetitions	Sequence Pause Time
6	BEADGC	1 time softly	20+ seconds

Play the multi-note sequence above and then let the vibrations slowly dissipate as you chant from your tradition. Then quietly clear the bowls on your side so the client can roll to her side and get up when she is ready. The closing procedure is shared with the client at the beginning of the session so she can simply get up at her convenience.

Clearing the Chakras

Approximately 30 minutes

This is a technique for clearing five of the seven internal energy chakra points—root, sacral, solar plexus, heart, and throat. For this therapy, you will place five bowls on the client's back, using the bowls as vibrational support for each other to clear the circulation of energy.

Client Positioning

Ask the client to lie on her stomach on the floor, face down, with knees and feet together. Her arms and hands can be by her sides, under her head, or however is most comfortable for her. For the client's comfort, have pillows nearby to place under her feet, chest, or stomach. You can sit by the client's hip on either the right or left side.

Bowl Placement

When placing each bowl in its respective position as follows, focus your healing intentions through the healing touch of your hand.

F on the backs of the knees
B on the floor above the head (no healing touch required)
C on the back of the sacrum
G on the back of the solar plexus
D on the back of the heart

Place the **A** and **E** bowls where you can reach them easily at the end of each part of the therapy.

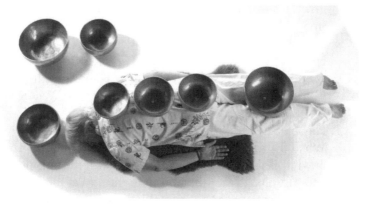

Bowl placement for clearing the chakras.

Striking the Bowls

For this therapy you'll be using both a cloth-covered striker and the pinky side of your fist.

Play the bowl softly, waiting several seconds between each strike of the bowl in the following sequences. After completing a sequence, allow the vibrations to dissipate 20+ seconds before moving to the next sequence in the list. *As much as possible, go slowly and keep the sound going throughout the therapy.*

Clearing the Internal Energy Points

1. Play the **F** bowl on the back of the client's knees six (6) times, waiting 5-10 seconds between each strike.
2. Play **F** and wait 3 seconds. Then play **C** on the sacrum and wait 5-10 seconds. Play this sequence 6 times. Wait 20+ seconds.
3. Play **F** and wait 3 seconds. Then play **G** on the solar plexus and wait 5-10 seconds. Play this sequence 6 times. Wait 20+ seconds.
4. Play **F** and wait 3 seconds. Then play **D** on the heart and wait 5-10 seconds. Play this sequence 6 times. Wait 20+ seconds.
5. Pick up the **A** bowl. Make a fist of your striker hand using the pad along the pinky side of your fist and strike the bowl. The **A** bowl doesn't touch the body. Move the bowl from side to side, directing the vibrations into the area at the base of the skull and along the neck. When the sound has dissipated, strike the **F** bowl. Repeat 3 times.
6. Play **F** and wait 3 seconds. Then play **B** above the head and wait 5-10 seconds. Play this sequence 6 times. Wait 20+ seconds.
7. Play **B** above the head 6 times.
8. When the sound has dissipated, pick up the **E** bowl. The **E** bowl doesn't touch the body. Strike it with the outside of your fist. Direct the vibrations into the area at the base of the skull and along the neck. When the sound has dissipated, strike the **F** bowl. Repeat 3 times.

Grounding the Internal Energy Points

In this section of the procedure you will remove the bowls from the client's body when the sound has dissipated, using a technique of consciously rolling the bottom of the bowl to one side as you gently lift the weight of the bowl off the body.

1. Play the **B** above the head and wait 3 seconds. Then play **D** and wait 5-10 seconds. Play this sequence 6 times. Wait 20+ seconds. Remove the **D** bowl.
2. Play **B** and wait 3 seconds. Then play **G** on the solar plexus and wait 5-10 seconds. Play this sequence 6 times. Wait 20+ seconds. Remove the bowl.
3. Play **B** and wait 3 seconds. Then play **C** on the sacrum and wait 5-10 seconds. Play this sequence 6 times. Wait 20+ seconds. Remove the **C** bowl.
4. Play **B** and wait 3 seconds. Then play **F** on the back of the knees and wait 5-10 seconds. Play this sequence 6 times. Wait 20+ seconds.
5. Play **F** and wait 3 seconds. Play this 6 times. Wait 20+ seconds. Remove the **F** bowl.

Stress and Depression Therapy

Approximately 30-45 minutes

This is a therapy for removing stress, giving peace, and relieving depression. This treatment can serve as a single stand alone healing session.

Client Positioning

Ask the client to lie on his stomach, on a properly prepared floor area. This might be a clean rug covered with a clean natural fiber sheet or blanket. For the client's comfort, have pillows nearby to place under his feet, chest, or stomach.

Have the client position his legs and feet so they are touching. His arms will lay comfortably 6-12" away from his body with palms facing up. The client will hold a bowl in each palm, so if weak, tender or inflexible wrists are a concern, have some small wash cloths available to bolster the weight and position of the bowls. You can sit on either the right or left side of the client, depending on your dominant side or the room layout.

Bowl Placement and Setup

When placing each bowl in its respective position as follows, focus your healing intentions through the healing touch of your hand. First, place one hand on the client at the placement site, being mindful of neutrality and client comfort with touch at sexually sensitive areas. This is a brief transfer of healing touch energy through the one hand as the other hand quickly but gently transfers the weight of the bowl onto the placement position.

F on the backs of the knees
B on the floor above the head (no healing touch required)
G on the palm of the client's right hand. (If the client's wrists are sensitive or inflexible, you may not want to use a big bowl.)
D on the palm of the client's left hand

Place the **A** and **E** bowls where you can reach them easily at the end of each part of the therapy. You will also need a tingsha close by.

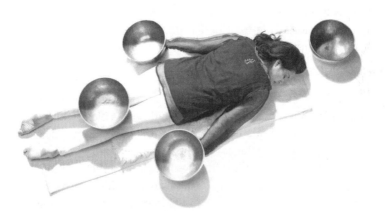

Bowl placement for stress and depression therapy.

Striking the Bowls

In this therapy you'll be using both a cloth or felt covered striker and your fist. There are five distinct parts to this treatment with four transitional steps between each of the parts. *As much as possible, go slowly and keep the sound going throughout the therapy.*

PART 1: Softly play the four bowls in the sequence **FBGD.** You may also go around clockwise or counterclockwise. Wait 5-10 seconds between each bowl, and allow the vibrations to dissipate for 20+ seconds after each sequence. Repeat the sequence of **FBGD** 4 times. Wait 20+ seconds.

After playing Part 1 above, play the tingsha lightly back and forth around the nape of the client's neck at the cranial sacral point. At the same time as the tingsha moves from side to side, cupping the nape of the neck, rotate the tingsha discs in small inward circles to create a pulsating healing vibration. Still rotating the tingsha, hold it approximately 2-4" above the client's body as you apply this pulsating vibration down to the base of the spine, and then back up to the nape of the neck. Finally, shift the tingsha to your left hand until it stops ringing.

PART 2: Play the four bowls in the sequence **FBGD.** You may also go around clockwise or counterclockwise. Wait 5-10 seconds between each bowl, and wait 20+ seconds after each sequence. Repeat the sequence of **FBGD** 4 times. Wait 20+ seconds.

After playing Part 2 above, pick up the **A** bowl and strike it with the outside of your closed fist to create a gentle resonance. Hold the bowl near the client's head at the base of their skull, moving the bowl left to right in a curved path, cupping the cranial sacral point.

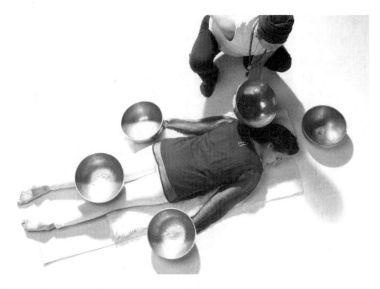

Hold the bowl near the client's head at the base of their skull.

PART 3: Play the four bowls in the sequence **FBGD**. You may also go around clockwise or counterclockwise. Wait 5-10 seconds between each bowl, waiting 20+ seconds after each sequence. Repeat the sequence of **FBGD** 4 times. Wait 20+ seconds.

After playing Part 3 above, play the tingsha lightly back and forth around the nape of the client's neck, cupping the cranial sacral point. At the same time as the tingsha moves from side to side around the nape of the neck, rotate the tingsha discs in small inward circles to create a pulsating healing vibration. Still rotating the tingsha, hold them approximately 2-4" above the client's body as apply this pulsating vibration down to the base of the spine, and then back up to the nape of the neck. Finally, shift the tingsha to your left hand, holding it until it stops ringing.

PART 4: Play the four bowls in the sequence **FBGD**. You may also go around clockwise or counterclockwise. Wait 5-10 seconds between each bowl, waiting 20+ seconds after each sequence. Repeat the sequence of **FBGD** 4 times. Wait 20+ seconds.

After playing Part 4 above, pick up the **E** bowl and strike it with the outside of your closed fist to create a gentle resonance. Hold the bowl near the client's head at the base of their skull, gently circling and rotating the bowl left to right in a curved path, cupping the cranial sacral point. With the bowl still resonating, take the bowl down the spine to just below the tailbone, then return back to the client's head. Repeat 2 more times.

PART 5: Play the four bowls in the sequence **FBGD**. You may also go around clockwise or counterclockwise. Wait 5-10 seconds between each bowl, waiting 20+ seconds after each sequence. Repeat the sequence of **FBGD** 4 times. Wait 20+ seconds.

When the healing vibrations have dissipated, hit the **B** bowl once softly and as the sound fades, remove the **G** and **D** palm bowls by consciously rolling the bottom of the bowl to one side as you gently lift the weight of the bowl off. Continue to play the **B** bowl several times, pausing at least 5 seconds between the strikes. Remove the **F** bowl from the back for the client's knees and set it on the floor below but not touching the client's feet. Play the bowl several more times.

To complete this therapy, remove the **G** and **D** bowls from the client's left and right hands. Remove the **F** bowl from between the knees and place it between the feet without touching them.

1. Play **F** and wait 3 seconds. Then play **B** above the head and wait 5-10 seconds. Play this sequence 6 times. Wait 20+ seconds.
2. Play **B** above the head 6 times.
3. Pick up the **F** bowl. Strike it with the outside of your fist. As the healing vibrations dissipate, move the bowl back and forth from side to side of the cranial sacral point at the nape of the client's neck. During this process continue playing the **F** bowl.

Removing the Bowls

It's important to note that when removing bowls from the client's hands and knees, they should be lifted off very carefully and not abruptly. Lift the bowl off slowly and at an angle.

Therapy to Ease Anger, Aggression, Arthritis, and High Blood Pressure

Client Positioning

The client should lie on his stomach on a rug on the floor. I suggest having pillows available to place under the client as needed for his comfort. The client should lie face down with knees and feet close together and arms in whatever position is comfortable for him. You will sit to the left of the client near his left hip.

Be sure when arranging the session with the client to instruct him to wear comfortable clothing free of exposed metal, zippers, belts, and jewelry.

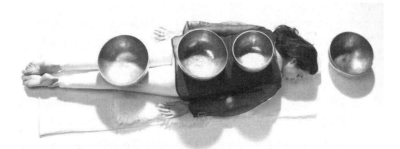

Bowl placement for the therapy to ease anger (the G bowl is not shown).

Bowl Placement and Setup

Place the singing bowls as follows:

F on the back of the client's knees
B above the client's head

C on the client's back over the sacrum

G near the client's left ear (rotating)

D on the client's back over the heart

After you have played the **C** bowl on the sacrum and **G** near the client's left ear you will reverse these bowls, playing the **G** bowl on the client's back over the solar plexus and the **C** bowl by his left ear.

Striking the Bowls

There are five parts (with four middle parts) to this chakra balancing therapy.

1. Play **FCDB** 4 times.

   Pick up the **G** bowl near the clients left ear and play it by hitting it with your closed fist to make it resonate. Rotate it around the base of the client's skull then go down the along client's spine and over the buttocks and back up the spine.

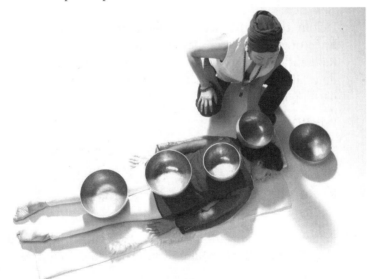

Rotating the G bowl around the base of the skull.

2. Play **BDCF** 4 times

Pick up the **G** bowl near the client's left ear and play it by hitting it with your closed fist to make it resonate. Rotate it around the base of the client's skull then go down along the client's spine and over the buttocks and back up the spine.

Exchange the **C** and **G** bowls placing the **G** bowl over the solar plexus area of the client's back. Place the **C** bowl near the client's left ear.

3. Play **FGDB** 4 times

Pick up the **C** bowl near the client's left ear and play it by hitting it with your closed fist to make it resonate. Rotate it around the base of the client's skull then go down along the client's spine and over the buttocks and back up the spine.

4. Play **BDGF** 4 times.

Pick up the **C** bowl near the client's left ear and play it by hitting it with your closed fist to make it resonate. Rotate it around the base of the client's skull then go down along the client's spine and over the buttocks and back up the spine.

5. Play **BDGF** 4 times.

6. When the bowls are silent, remove the **D** bowl from the client's back. Wait 5-10 seconds.

7. Remove the **G** bowl from the client's back. Wait 5-10 seconds.

8. Remove the **F** bowl from the back of the client's knees and place it on the floor about 6 inches below the client's feet.

9. Play the **F** bowl several times slowly.

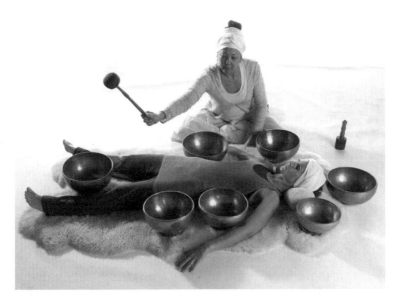

Prone posture therapy.

Prone Posture

Approximately 20-30 minutes

In this therapy, the client lies on his back on a floor or massage table, giving you access to the top of the head and the brain and allowing you to stimulate the third eye and the energy body.

You will need:
- An 8-12" diameter bowl that fits easily in one hand
- One large fabric-covered striking mallet
- One large leather-covered rubbing mallet
- Cushions and sticky pads for the bowls, if necessary
- A set of 7 bowls

1. Place the 7 bowls in their respective chakra positions around the client.
2. Strike the bowls in the sequence B, F, D, G, C, A, E in

quick succession with 3 seconds between each strike.
Once the sound dissipates completely, and there is a deep
state of shunyata in the silence, remove the crown chakra
bowl to prepare for the next step.

3. If you're using a table, stand in a grounded position with
   both feet solidly on the floor and feel your weight resting
   equally on your feet. Relax your jaw, face, and shoulders.
   Place your hands on either side of the client's head, with
   fingers flanking the ears, as shown, touching lightly. Your
   little and ring fingers are positioned below the ears while
   your middle and index fingers are positioned above the
   ears. Take 3 long breaths to center yourself, and bring
   your awareness to your contact with the client's head.
   Establish a rapport with the client's internal bodily
   rhythm. This step may take 2-3 minutes.

4. With the 8-12" bowl on your palm, strike it with the large
   fabric mallet, and holding it 3-4" from the client, move it
   from the forehead to the back of the head. As much as

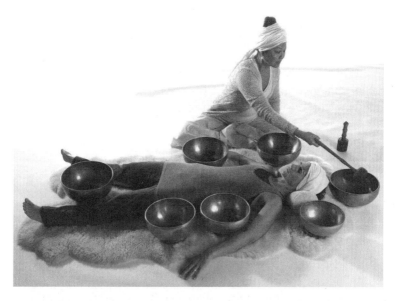

Prone posture therapy.

possible, have the sound come off the lip of the bowl by tipping it toward the head. This will take 20-30 seconds. Repeat this two times, then wait until the sound completely dissipates.

5. Strike the bowl on your palm again. Holding the bowl 3-4" from the client, move the bowl from ear to ear over the top of the head and back again, pausing above each ear 3 times, for a total of 6 passes over the top of the head. Replace the crown chakra bowl to prepare for the next step.

6. Strike the bowls around the client in the sequence F, B, D, G, C, A, E in quick succession with 3 seconds between each strike. Repeat step 3 while the sound dissipates completely.

7. Repeat steps 4 and 5.

8. Strike the bowls around the client in the sequence F, C, G, D, A, E, B in quick succession with 3 seconds between each strike. Repeat step 3 while the sound dissipates completely. Remove the crown chakra bowl to prepare for the next step.

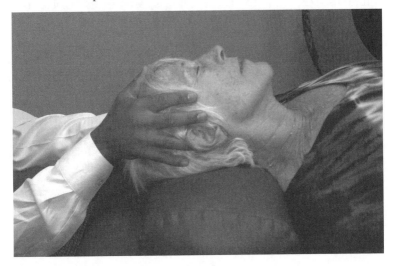

Prone posture therapy, step 3.

9. Repeat steps 4 and 5.

10. Repeat step 3 and note any changes in what you feel as you touch the client's head for a couple of minutes. You are looking for changes in the quality of the tissue, to see if it has softened and become more resilient. The client's breathing should also have slowed down and deepened. These are indications that the body is responding to the power of the sound vibration.

11. Softly strike the bowls as in step 8 to close.

Side Lying Posture (Nirvana)

Approximately 20-30 minutes

This therapy stimulates and harmonizes all the chakras, activates the energy body, and integrates the emotional body. The client is on the floor or a massage table on her side, with a pillow under her head. Her legs are bent with a bolster positioned between them. It is generally easier to work on a massage table because some areas of the body are more accessible. Stand behind the client so you can reach the entire spine and feet. If you're working on the floor, kneel behind the client, and to make the bowls easier to reach, place the A and G bowls at the client's back along with the others, in this order: B, E, A, D, G, C, F.

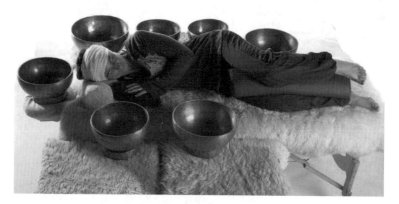

Side lying posture therapy, client positioning.

You will need:

- An 8-12" diameter bowl of any note
- One large fabric-covered striking mallet
- One 1.5"-3" diameter leather covered rubbing mallet
- One bolster for legs and pillow for the head
- A set of bowls. Note: If you only have one 8-12" bowl, you can still use this technique by omitting steps 2, 8, and 10.

1. Place the 7 bowls in their respective chakra positions around the client.
2. Strike the bowls in the sequence B, F, D, G, C, A, E in quick succession with 3 seconds between each strike. Once the sound dissipates completely, and there is a deep state of shunyata in the silence, remove the crown chakra bowl to prepare for the next step.
3. If you're using a table, stand in a grounded position with both feet solidly on the floor and feel your weight resting equally on your feet. Relax your jaw, face, and shoulders. Place one hand on the back of the head and the other on the small of the back, touching lightly. Take 3 long breaths to center yourself, and bring your awareness to your contact with the client's head. Establish a rapport with the client's internal bodily rhythm. This step may take 2-3 minutes.
4. Holding the 8-12" bowl on the palm of one hand, rub or strike the bowl at a distance of 3-4" from the body at the base of the client's head. Slowly move the bowl down the spine, pausing at the small of the back, and hold for 5 seconds.
5. Move the bowl to the tailbone and allow it to resonate the whole lower portion of the body. Hold it there for 5 seconds. You may need to strike the bowl again when moving to the tailbone if the resonance is too soft.
6. Move the bowl to the soles of the feet and hold it there for 5 seconds. You may need to strike the bowl again when

moving to the feet if the resonance is too soft.

7. Finally, move the bowl slowly to the base of the head.
8. Strike the bowls around the client in the sequence F, B, D, G, C, A, E in quick succession with 3 seconds between each strike. Repeat step 3 while the sound dissipates completely. Remove the crown chakra bowl to prepare for the next step.
9. Repeat steps 3-7.
10. Strike the bowls around the client in the sequence F, C, G, D, A, E, B in quick succession with 3 seconds between each strike. Repeat step 3 while the sound dissipates completely. Remove the crown chakra bowl to prepare for the next step.
11. Repeat steps 3-7.
12. Repeat step 3 and note any changes in what you feel as you touch the client for a couple of minutes. You are looking for changes in the quality of the tissue, to see if it has softened and become more resilient. The client's breathing should also have slowed down and deepened. These are

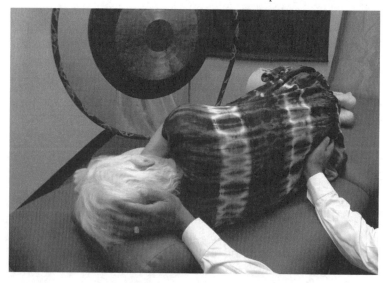

Side lying posture therapy, step 3, hand positioning without bowls.

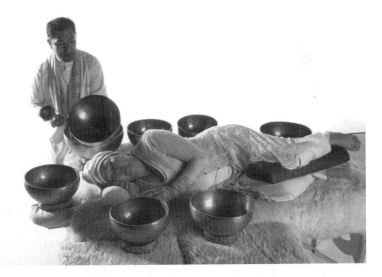

Side lying posture therapy, step 4.

indications that the body is responding to the power of
the sound vibration.

13. Softly strike the bowls as in step 8 to close.

This whole sequence can be repeated on the other side for an
additional 20-30 minutes.

Healing the Head, Spine and Feet

Approximately 10 to 15 minutes

This is a very advanced healing treatment known for its effectiveness in releasing stress and tension in the spine, head and feet.
This method is also helpful in curing insomnia, migraine headaches,
and muscle tension.

It requires 4 large bowls and a stool for the client to sit on. The
first bowl goes on top of the stool, the client's feet are placed inside
a second bowl and a third bowl is inverted on their head, while the
practitioner strikes a fourth large bowl to treat the front, back and
sides of the head.

You will repeat a sequence of steps 3 times within a 10-15 minute timeframe. However, you may let your intuition guide you as to whether you should extend the time by repeating the sequence again or concentrating on an area.

You will need:
- One approximately 14" diameter bowl to place on the client's stool
- One 16+" diameter bowl for the client to place their feet in
- One extra large fabric covered striking mallet to be used for the stool bowl and the foot bowl
- Two 9-12" diameter bowls: one for the client's head and one for you to apply vibration around the client's head
- One approximately 4" donut cushion for the head bowl or a piece of non-slip pad
- One large fabric covered striking mallet, to be used for the head bowl and the practitioner's fourth bowl.
- One round stool approximately 14-16" high, depending on the size of your client's body. Ideally, when seated, the thighs should be parallel to the floor and not slanted. This provides a good ergonomic position for the client, in particular providing a neutral position for their lower back.
- 1 or 2 large donut cushions approximately 6" in diameter. You may need the additional donut cushion to raise the stool bowl up higher.

1. Place one or both of the 6" donut cushions on the stool and then place the inverted stool bowl on top of the cushion(s). Place the foot bowl in front of the stool where the client will sit. The height of the stool bowl should be equal to the length of the client's lower leg so that their upper thigh is parallel with the floor when they are seated.
2. Getting your client into seated position on the stool is an important part of a successful treatment. Have the client begin by standing with one foot on either side of the large foot bowl. Assist her in sitting on the stool and then take

note of the stool bowl's position when her full weight is on it. Check that the bowl is balanced and not sagged down or tilted onto the stool, which will dampen the healing vibrations. You may need to ask her to stand up for adjustments and then sit again to reappraise the stool bowl's position. Make any adjustments needed, then have her gently sit down, checking with her to confirm that she feels balanced, strong and secure.

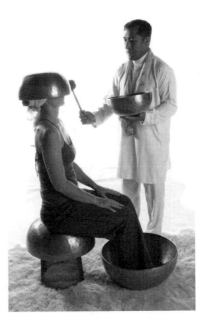

Healing the head, spine and feet therapy: step 5.

Now, ask her to move one foot into the larger foot bowl, followed by the second foot.

3. Now ask her to sit up straight with her chest lifted and her hands resting in her lap. Her back should be perpendicular to the floor. Let her know that she should expect a cushion and bowl to be placed on her head. First, place the 4" donut cushion on her head, then invert the large head bowl and place it on top of the cushion. Be sure it's balanced and comfortable! Ask her to close her eyes and take long deep breaths during this treatment.

4. Stand at either her right or left side with the other 9-12" bowl positioned nearby so you can easily access it later in this treatment.

5. Use your non-dominant hand to rest one or two fingers on top of the inverted bowl on the client's head to steady it.

Then, gently hit the side of the head bowl with the large fabric covered mallet using a downward striking motion. Wait twenty seconds for the vibrations to dissipate and then strike the head bowl at the back side of the head. Wait 20 seconds until the vibrations dissipate and then finally, strike the bowl on the other side of the head. Immediately move to the next step.

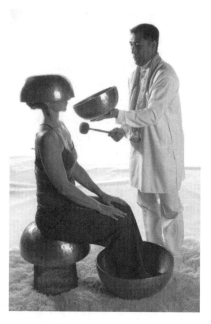

Healing the head, spine and feet therapy: step 9.

6. Now take the extra large fabric covered mallet and strike the stool bowl firmly 3 times in rapid succession to bring up a deep vibration. Make sure to strike within 2" of the rim of the bowl and take special caution so you don't hit your client's leg with the striker! Move immediately to the next step.

7. Still using the extra large fabric covered mallet, strike the foot bowl 3 times in rapid succession. Now wait for all the bowl vibrations to dissipate.

8. Repeat step 5.

9. Immediately pick up the 9-12" bowl that you set aside and hold it in the flat palm of your non-dominant hand. Strike it either by fist or with the large mallet and then move it to the throat chakra. Next slowly move the bowl downward to the heart chakra while it's still vibrating. Now, slowly move the bowl downward to the sacral chakra and strike it

again. Pause a few seconds, and changing the direction of movement, slowly move the bowl upward to an inch below the head bowl, slightly overlapping the inside space of the head bowl. This will create a sound chamber as the vibrations of the two bowls interact and create a soothing space around the client's head. Be very careful that the two bowls do not touch. If they do, it will create a highly disturbing, jarring noise that is extremely irritating to the client and disruptive to the healing. Wait until the vibrations completely dissipate. Put aside the bowl in your hand.

10. Repeat steps 5, 6, and 7.

11. Immediately pick up the bowl you set aside and hold it in the flat palm of your non-dominant hand. Strike it either by fist or with the large mallet and then move it from the back of the throat chakra down to the tail bone at the base of the spine. At the tail bone, strike it again and then slowly move it up to the back of the head just beneath the rim of the head bowl, overlapping slightly but not touching, as you did in step 9. After pausing 2 seconds, move the bowl around to the left ear and then around to the right ear, repeating until the sound dissipates.

12. Repeat steps 5, 6, and 7. Wait for all the vibrations to dissipate and then gently remove the head bowl. Next ask her to take her feet out of the large foot bowl, placing one foot on either side of the bowl on the floor. Then assist her in standing up and moving away from the foot bowl.

Healing with the Tingsha

Ear Therapy

Approximately 3-5 minutes

This treatment is for hearing problems in children as well as adults. You can use either the tingsha or a small singing bowl.

Client Positioning

Ask the client to sit either in a chair or cross legged on the floor in a meditation posture.

Choosing the Tingsha

An approximately 3" diameter tingsha is usually best for healing. Select a tingsha with a pleasant tone and longer resonance.

Striking the Tingsha

Remember that the ear is delicate. Strike the tingsha approximately 24" away from the client's head. As soon as you strike it, bring it quickly within 2-3" of the client's ear, hold in that position for approximately 5 seconds, and then slowly bring it back to where you started. Repeat this procedure for about 3-5 minutes.

If you're using a singing bowl instead, just follow the same procedure as you would with tingsha, striking the bowl with a leather-covered or felt-covered mallet.

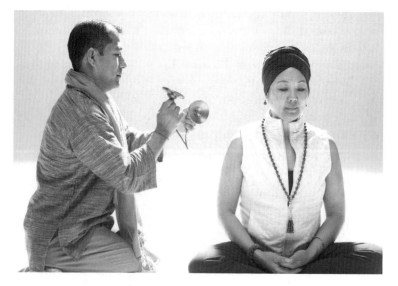

Using the tingsha in ear therapy.

Using Crystals with the Bowls

CRYSTALS are very powerful for healing. You can place a crystal on a non-slip piece of mesh inside your singing bowl. The kind of flexible plastic mesh you use to line a kitchen drawer is good for this purpose. It's best to use a large crystal so that it won't topple over when the bowl is hit (ideally, larger than the one in the following photograph).

Each chakra has a color and corresponding crystals associated with it. Use the following chart to help you choose the appropriate crystals to use for healing each chakra.

Chakra	Color	Crystals
1st	red	ruby, garnet, jasper
2nd	orange	bloodstone, orange calcite, carnelian
3rd	yellow, yellow-green	amber, citrine, malachite,
4th	pink, green	rose quartz, agate, emerald, jade, aventurine, dioptase
5th	blue	moonstone, aquamarine, sapphire, turquoise, kayanite
6th	dark blue	diamond, sodalite, lapis lazuli, smoky quartz, angelite
7th	purple	amethyst, ametrine, apophyllite, prehnite

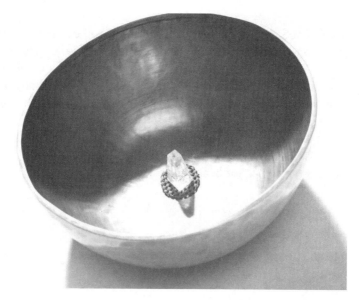

Using a crystal in a singing bowl.

Puja – A Prosperity Practice

PUJA addresses prosperity on many levels—from relationships to finances, feng shui, removing negative energy, and manifesting aspirations. Puja is also a prayer for the welfare of others or for the favorable results of an undertaking in business or personal life. You may also honor ancestors or loved ones who have passed on, asking the Divine to bring their souls to peace and rest.

How to do it? First, purify yourself with a shower or bath. Dress yourself in clean clothes, being careful to avoid the use of any leather objects such as belts, shoes, or wallets. This is a tradition based on avoiding the suffering of sentient beings. Optimally, you should be barefooted, though you may choose to wear socks.

Many items and elements can be included in your personal puja, which is done in your sacred altar room. Water is the most important. This is what you will need:

- Small container for water
- Altar table with pictures of statues of ancestors, guru, deities, guides, etc.

- Bell, gong, or singing bowls
- Incense, holder, and matches
- Vase with flower(s)
- Small spoon
- Fruit offerings

Once clean and dressed, take the water container and fill it with water, holding a very sacred intention for its use as blessed water that will cleanse and sanctify. Bring it to your sacred altar and spoon a few drops onto the statues or at the base of the picture frames with the intention of giving the gift of fresh water to honor your teachers.

Next, light the incense and offer the smoke of the incense to your teachers as you move your hand in a clockwise motion. With the other hand ring the bell, gong, or singing bowl. The sound of the bell removes negative energy in your house and it brings your consciousness to the present moment. During this time, chant your mantra or focus your intention to manifest your soul's wish. Now, place the incense in the incense holder.

The impact of this water ceremony is very important and you may wish to use the flower dipped in the holy water to sprinkle cleansing water drops around the room if there's been a particularly negative energy present. When you sprinkle the water, it removes any unseen negative forces. Once a month, quarter, half year, or year this house cleansing can be done.

Because the holy water is sacred, it will sit on your altar the remainder of the day and night. The next morning you may wish to pour any unused amounts onto a plant before getting fresh water for the new day.

Only one person in a household needs to observe puja for the household to benefit from this prosperity practice.

Using Singing Bowls
with Other Healing Modalities

SOME massage therapists find that it is useful to give their patients singing bowl therapy before a massage to speed up the relaxation process. Similarly, some acupuncturists and chiropractors use singing bowl treatments as part of their practice to amplify the effects of their work.

Greg Storozuk of Labyrinths of Colorado uses singing bowls in his labyrinth experiences:

> To enhance and heighten the labyrinth experience, singing bowls with the commensurate chakra tone may be placed at each turn and struck by the walker before entering and when leaving each respective pathway. Another method would be to position bowl keepers at the top and sides of the labyrinth, striking the bowls with the appropriate chakra note, or striking the C, E, and G notes to form a pleasant chord surrounding the walker.

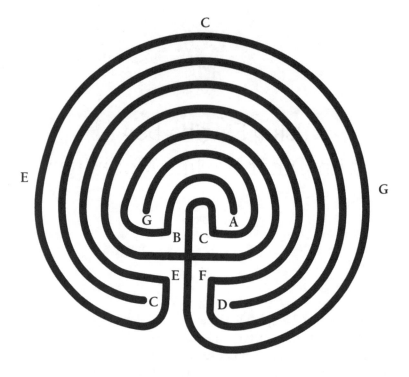

Bowl placement in a labyrinth

Acknowledgements

MANY spiritual teachers have come along in my life—some for a few hours, some for many days while in retreat, and some every time I needed them. Those for whom I have especially deep respect are the ones who are keeping alive the art of sound and vibration healing, with shamanic drums, gongs, or singing bowls. The use of singing bowls in particular is a dying healing art back in Nepal.

Being born as part of two great cultures was a wonderful advantage for me. I was born in a small village called Khandabari in Nepal. Buddhism and Hinduism are the two major cultures we have in my village and in the surrounding villages of walking distance. I would like to acknowledge and thank all healers, lamas, monks, pundits, gurus, bijuwas, shamans, jakri, and Ayurvedic medicine men. I would especially like to thank the following wonderful teachers that I have met along the way:

Great teacher Master Dorje Thingo of Kimathanka (a very remote village that borders Tibet), known as a medicine man with Ayurvedic knowledge. He is also known as a great lama and a teacher of the power of intention. He says sound is the medium, and we bring forth positive healing energy through our intention.

Jejen Lama from Namachhe (not Solu Khumbu's Namache Bazar), sound and vibrational healer. He is also known as a master in mantra chanting. In his healing ceremonies he chants mantras, uses Tibetan sage incense, shakes his body, and blows on the body part that needs to be healed.

I would like to thank my village friend, Umang Bhotia's uncle Nang Ritar Lama, who lives in Chamtang. He uses the cymbal (ting-sha) for healing.

I would also like to thank my spiritual teacher H.H. Acharya Shree 108 Tahal Kishor Maharaj. I am grateful to him for differentiating between the Vedic chakra system and the Tibetan chakra system.

In addition, I want to thank my brother and sister-in-law, Narayan Shrestha and Shreejana Shrestha, for bringing me to America.

My colleagues in sound and vibrational healing have touched my life and I am grateful to them.

I would like to thank Lee Veal and my spiritual sisters Cynthia Cunningham and Donna Wong, who have been enormous help in compiling the material for this book.

Thanks to Dr. Andrew Fryer for writing the foreword.

I would like to thank Connie Shaw for her editing; Gina Martinez for modeling, taking photos, and doing Photoshop work; Donna Wong, Cathryn Cunningham, Trishul, Paul Foerster, Rachel Hildebrandt, and Nathan Tomaszewski for posing for photographs; Charles and Debbie Imstepf, Wendy Cima, and Kati Walker for their photography; and Dave Watson for his Photoshop work.

Last but not least, I would like to thank my wife Ruby Shrestha and my daughter Sarina Shrestha simply for being part of my life.

PHOTOGRAPHY AND DRAWING CREDITS

www.imstepf.com: title page, pages 14, 16, 20, 31 (top), 34, 35, 36, 37, 38, 39, 40 (bottom), 43, 48, 50, 51, 53, 55, 58, 59, 61, 63, 65, 84, 89, 90, 93, 96, 98, 100, 101, 103, 104, 106, 109, 111, 112, 114, 116, 124

Gina Martinez: pages 105, 108

Kati Walker: page 72

Suren Shrestha: pages 28, 29, 40 (top), 42

Wendy Cima: front cover, pages 31 (bottom), 44, 47, 52, 76, 77, 78, 79, 80, 81, 85, 86, 88, 92

All drawings by Suren Shrestha, Photoshop work by David Watson and Gina Martinez

ABOUT THE AUTHOR

Suren Shrestha was born in Nepal, about forty-five miles southeast of Mt. Everest. In the village where he grew up, people were healed by herbalists, monks, and medicine men using shaman's drums, gongs, and mantras. He came to the United States as a teenager, later attended college, and received a B.S. in Civil Engineering. Noting the growing interest in alternative medicine in the U.S., Suren returned to Nepal to learn how to practice ancient healing techniques that use sound and vibration. Suren has given workshops and assisted clients with healing bowl work internationally. He is raising funds through his teaching to build the Aama Orphanage School for children in his native village, and is donating all his proceeds from the sale of this book to the project. He lives in Boulder, Colorado, with his wife and daughter, where he teaches singing bowl therapies at his school, Atma Buti Sound and Vibrational School (atmabuti.org).

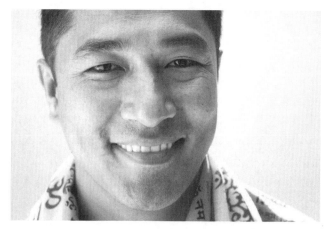

Sentient Publications, LLC publishes books on cultural creativity, experimental education, transformative spirituality, holistic health, new science, ecology, and other topics, approached from an integral viewpoint. Our authors are intensely interested in exploring the nature of life from fresh perspectives, addressing life's great questions, and fostering the full expression of the human potential. Sentient Publications' books arise from the spirit of inquiry and the richness of the inherent dialogue between writer and reader.

Our Culture Tools series is designed to give social catalyzers and cultural entrepreneurs the essential information, technology, and inspiration to forge a sustainable, creative, and compassionate world.

We are very interested in hearing from our readers. To direct suggestions or comments to us, or to be added to our mailing list, please contact:

SENTIENT PUBLICATIONS, LLC

PO Box 7204
Boulder, CO 80306
303-443-2188
contact@sentientpublications.com
www.sentientpublications.com